Tibetan Medicine Series
363EN

FIRST INTEGRATIVE MEDICINE

CONFERENCE

Mental Disorders and Dementia:
A Dialogue Between Conventional, Homeopathic, Tibetan, and Chinese Medicines

BARCELONA, SPAIN

January 2014

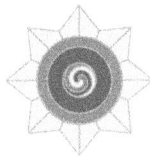

ཡེ་ཤེས་ཝོ་གྲུབ་ཅིན་ཀྱི་འཁར་ལེ་ག།
Shang Shung Publications

This volume contains the proceedings of the presentations given at the
First Integrative Medical Conference
held at Casal del Médico,
Via Laietana, 10, Barcelona, Spain
January 10-12, 2014

Conference Organizers:
THE INTERNATIONAL SHANG SHUNG INSTITUTE
THE INTERNATIONAL DZOGCHEN COMMUNITY

Collaborators:
AMCP (Associazione per la Medicina Centrata sulla Persona – ONLUS – ENTE
MORALE)

Sponsors:
FUNDACIÓ ENRIC MIRALLE
SANTIVERI (nutrición y vida)

Cover design: Yuchen Namkhai
Photo: Gino Vitiello

ISBN: 9978-88-7834-141-8

Conference Schedule

Friday, January 10, 2014 * 4:00pm-8:15pm
Introduction to Integrative Medicine

Saturday, January 11, 2014 * 10:00am-1:45pm / 4:00pm-7:15pm
Mental Disorders

Sunday, January 12, 2014 * 10:00am-2:15pm
Dementia

This publication has been realized thanks to the voluntary work of many people from the International Dzogchen Community. Our heartfelt thanks go to them all.

A special thanks to our teacher Chögyal Namkhai Norbu.

Contents

Conference Organizers

The **International Shang Shung Institute** is dedicated to the preservation and study of Tibetan language, medicine, culture, and traditions. It has centers in Italy, Russia, the United States, the United Kingdom, Argentina, Australia, Austria, and the Netherlands.

The **International Dzogchen Community** is a nonprofit organization whose members are dedicated to the study and practice of Dzogchen, the highest teaching of the Tibetan spiritual traditions. Transmitted in an unbroken lineage of spiritual masters over many generations, the knowledge of Dzogchen encourages each of us to increase presence and awareness in our daily lives. As a direct consequence, it can meaningfully contribute to the evolution of a more harmonious, caring, and collaborative society.

The **School of Tibetan Medicine** (USA) of the Shang Shung Institute is the first school of Tibetan medicine in the West to offer a full, four-year course of study following the traditional curriculum. The school also offers specialized complementary courses taught by guest professors on a number of related subjects.

Moderators' Biographies

Ms. Eloísa Álvarez Centeno holds a degree in psychology from the University of Barcelona. She also holds a master's degree in humanistic integrative psychotherapy from the Erich Fromm Institute and is a member of the Humanistic Integrative Psychotherapy Association (Asociación de Piscoterapia Integradora Humanista or APIH) and of the Spanish Federation of Psychotherapist Associations (Federación Española de Asociaciones de Piscoterapeutas or FEAP).

She is a graduate of the International Institute for Bioenergetic Analysis (IIBA) as a bioenergetic analyst (TPC) and studied integrative psychotherapy as part of the SAT Program with Dr. Claudio Naranjo.

She currently offers individual and couples psychotherapy, but also has experience in child psychotherapy, adolescent psychotherapy, and group psychotherapy.

Dr. Eva Juan Linares holds a degree in clinical psychology, is a psycho-oncology specialist and a doctor in health and learning psychology. She is currently head of the Psycho-Oncology Unit at the Santa Creu i Sant Pau Hospital in Barcelona and an associate professor of psychology and nursing at the Autonomous University of Barcelona (UAB).

Dr. Tomás Álvaro Naranjo has a doctorate in medicine and surgery and a degree in clinical psychology. He is an expert in psychoneuroimmunology and in energy psychology techniques. He has studied extensively in the field of bioenergetic and vibrational medicine. He is currently the director of the Arjuna Tortosa Integrative Medicine Center.

Dr. María Carmen Martínez Tomás holds a degree in medicine and surgery from the University of Barcelona. She is a homoeopathic health practitioner and has a degree in homoeopathy from L'Ecole d'Étude d'Homéopathie, Association pour l'enseignement post-universitarie de l'Homéopathie in Geneva. She is a professor for the master's degree program in traditional medicine and nursing at the University of Barcelona and the Autonomous University of Barcelona. She is a professor for the master's degree program in oncology nursing at the Sant Pau Hospital and the Autonomous University of Barcelona.

Dr. Tomás teaches ongoing training courses as part of the training plan of the Official School of Nursing in Barcelona (COIB), where she gives classes on emotional self-management, Ho'oponopono, and metamorphic technique. She is a professor of the International School of Forgiveness based in Italy.

She is author of *HO'OPONOPONO, lo siento, perdóname, te amo* (HO'OPONOPONO: I'm Sorry, Forgive Me, I Love You) and *El Espíritu de Aloha: El poder de ser feliz ahora* (The Aloha Spirit: The Power of Being Happy Now), both published by Oceano-Ambar.

She set up the Círculos de Sanación con Ho'oponopono (Ho'oponopono Healing Circles) in Spain – supported worldwide via the Ho'oponopono Network of Agartam, a nonprofit group of persons.

Foreword

The aim of this three-day event, the first Integrative Medicine Conference in Barcelona, Spain, was to find a meeting point between the various medical disciplines present in the cultures of our planet: Western medicine, both homeopathic and allopathic, and Eastern medicine, in particular Tibetan and Chinese medicine. Although their theoretical base and technical tools are different, all of these disciplines have as their common aim the person's health in all its various aspects. A dialogue and comparison without preconceptions should be an enriching encounter for all.

In his book *Birth, Life and Death*, Chögyal Namkhai Norbu gives us a clear vision of the concept of medicine in the Tibetan medical tradition: "The human body is the basis or root of medical science... Our basic nature is not a figure of speech but constitutes the foundation of the concrete and real condition of our body and, as such, warrants the focused attention of every living human being."

He also explains how Tibetan medicine sees the role of the doctor, and how ancient texts describe six qualifications or necessary causes for undertaking the medical profession: capacity, meaning knowledge of medicine; good intentions, thoughts aimed at the good of others; commitment, specifically to help the sick; attention, being accurate, not imprecise; diligence, dedication to one's work; and availability, being open to the sick, attempting to understand their condition.

These six qualifications form the underpinning of what are called the six principles to be developed: openness to study in order to perfect the knowledge of medicine; desire to persevere in the commitment to medical practice; capacity to dedicate oneself totally to the sick and to face difficulties and uncomfortable conditions for their good; an attitude of justice and balance toward patients; commitment to develop one's own capacities to the full; and, finally, a profound knowledge of human nature.

The ancient texts also distinguish three kinds of doctor according to the results they achieve: the common doctor, who has not studied in great depth and is able to deal with illnesses on a material level only; the higher level doctor, who is expert in all medical techniques and knows how to act on the energetic conditions of the individual; and the supreme level doctor, who has attained full knowledge of human nature and knows how to cure the deepest causes of illness.

This last level is often reached by Tibetan doctors and is an ideal that everyone who works in this field should try to aim for, wherever they are in the world. It is clear that such a concept is in no way different from the objectives of Western medicine, both in the past (Greek and Roman medicine) and the present. Nor is it different from those of Chinese medicine.

The allopathic, homeopathic, Chinese, and Tibetan doctors who participated in this event all had similar approaches to the patient, with one and the same aim: to eliminate suffering from body, mind, and energy, using different techniques and applications arising from the cultural, social, economic, and spiritual evolution of their respective societies.

Most of the participants expressed a wish to see a common language created that would permit the integration implied by the term integrative medicine: an integration of concepts, knowledge, and tools useful in all cultures and traditions because they apply to the same reality, a person with a condition of health or of illness. This level of integration is a difficult objective, but we can achieve it if we concentrate our efforts on three main points: to create a comprehensive language that would allow us to communicate among the different disciplines; to create a series of protocols of intervention (common to all the various medical disciplines and drawing on the knowledge of each) in order to jointly confront the various problems people suffer from in their body, mind, energy, and spiritual life; to create an integrated medical facility so that these protocols can be applied in hospitals, rest homes, and medical and walk-in clinics.

If the days we shared in Barcelona can give us the possibility to create tools for communication and coordination, protocols, and data analysis, and if we are able to make our respective skill sets available to doctors of every tradition and discipline to help them to offer more effective service, it may well contribute to the understanding of the global humanity of the person, showing that illness is only a part of a person's whole self. That would be an extremely positive outcome.

Carlos Enrique Ramos
Venice, February 9, 2014

Introduction to Integrative Medicine

Friday, January 10, afternoon

(1st session)

Good evening ladies and gentlemen. Welcome to this first symposium of integrative medicine. This symposium is the result of a conference on Tibetan medicine held in La Laguna, Tenerife, in 2013, organized by the International Shang Shung Institute and by the International Dzogchen Community Cultural Association.

Shang Shung Institute, together with the International Dzogchen Community, has organized this symposium this year with the aim of opening the door to cooperation between various medical systems and approaches: conventional medicine, alternative or complementary medicine, such as homeopathy, and traditional medicine from ancient cultures, such as Tibetan medicine and Chinese medicine. So this marks the opening of a dialogue between specialists from various fields as part of an effort to promote and foster integrative medicine in an international framework. An example is the National Values Plan we are developing here in Catalonia and also other global initiatives we are going to be talking about during the symposium.

As you can see, we are presenting a highly interesting program with speakers from very different background who are going to speak about different topics in the framework of dementia and mental illnesses and disorders.

We hope that you will enjoy the symposium and would like to thank you for being here. Now we give the word to Ms. Eloisa Álvarez Centeno, the moderator for this afternoon.

Moderator: Ms. Eloisa Álvarez Centeno

Good afternoon. I am here to introduce the speakers of this afternoon who will also participate in the roundtable. First we will have Professor Chögyal Namkhai Norbu, followed by Doctor Phuntsog Wangmo.

Professor Emeritus Namkhai Norbu is President of the International Shang Shung Institute, of the International Dzogchen Community, and of the NGO A.S.I.A.

One of the foremost living Dzogchen masters, he was born in Derge, Tibet, in 1938. He studied at important monastic universities, completing the rigorous traditional course of study and receiving degrees in philosophy and literature and Tibetan medicine.

In 1955 he met Rigdzin Changchub Dorje (1863-1961), his principal Dzogchen teacher, whose lifestyle and way of teaching inspired him profoundly. From 1954 to 1957 he was instructor of Tibetan language at the University for Minorities in Cheng-Du, People's Republic of China.

In 1958, while in India, he worked as author and chief editor of Tibetan textbooks at the development office of the government of Sikkim, in the town of Gangtok. In 1960 started his academic collaboration with the well-known orientalist Professor G. Tucci, at ISMEO (Istituto per il Medio e Estremo Oriente – Institute of the Middle and Far East) in Rome, Italy.

From 1962 to 1992 he taught Tibetan language and literature at the Università degli Studi di Napoli "L'Orientale," the school of oriental studies at the University of Naples.

Namkhai Norbu has focused his research mainly on the ancient history of Tibet, thoroughly investigating the autochthonous pre-Buddhist tradition and the monarchic age connected to the Shang Shung kingdom. Other fields of his research have included the Tibetan nomad populations; the origin, theory, and practice of astrology; and Tibetan traditional medicine.

In addition to initiating and participating in the First Integrative Medicine Workshop at the Casal del Médico in Barcelona, Spain, in

2014, Namkhai Norbu has participated in important international congresses such as the First International Congress on Tibetan Medicine, Ca' Foscari University, Venice, Italy, 1983; the international seminar "Introduzione e storia della medicina tibetana" (Introduction and History of Tibetan Medicine), Santo Spirito Hospital, Rome, Italy, 1985; the Second International Congress on Tibetan Language, Siena University, Italy, 1992; the Third International Conference on Tibetan Language, Columbia University and Trace Foundation, New York, USA, 2011; the International Seminar on Tibetan Medicine and Culture, La Laguna University, Tenerife, Spain (2011, 2012, 2013); and a conference on "Tibetan Medicine as a Heritage for Humanity" in the Faculty of Medicine at the University of Bologna, Italy, 2012.

Parallel to his work as a university professor, Namkhai Norbu regularly gives retreat seminars on the Dzogchen teaching. In that context, he has been invited to participate in international events such as Spirit of Peace: 40 Years of the United Nations, Europaplein, Amsterdam, Holland, 1985. Inspired by Namkhai Norbu, a monument dedicated to peace was inaugurated in the town of Grosseto, Italy, in 1990.

Brief bibliography: *Journey Among the Tibetan Nomads*; *Drung Deu Bon*; *The Necklace of Zi*; *Zhang Zhung: Images from a Lost Kingdom*; *The Light of Kailash* (3 volumes); *A Practical Manual of Tibetan Moxibustion*; *The Practice of Tibetan Ku-Nye Massage*; *Yantra Yoga: The Tibetan Yoga of Movement*; *On Birth, Life and Death*; *The Art and Practice of Yantra Yoga*; and *The Crystal and the Way of Light*.

Namkhai Norbu has founded various organizations to promote the cultural heritage of Tibet, such as the International Shang Shung Institute, which works to preserve and disseminate Tibetan culture in the West, and A.S.I.A. (Association for International Solidarity in Asia), an NGO committed to cooperation and development not only in Asia but all over the world.

PRESENTATION

NAMKHAI NORBU
Total Integration: Beyond the Relative Health Condition

Good evening everybody.

I wish to thank the organizers for this meeting. I would also like to thank all the professors and doctors who are participating in this conference. We know that medicine is very important for human beings. Everybody needs health. If there is illness, we need medicine to cure it. Even if there is no problem, we need medicine for living healthy. This contribution comes from medicine and the work of doctors.

In general we distinguish between Western and Eastern medicine, which includes the Chinese, Tibetan, and Indian traditions among many others. But the real purpose of medicine is to cure human beings and help them feel better. For someone who has a serious illness, it does not really matter what kind of system or tradition their doctor follows, whether it is Western or Eastern; the only thing that counts is to overcome the problem. So when we work with medicine we should understand that. That is something very important. The first thing is to not remain limited.

Another crucial factor is that we need to understand the condition of the individual. In general, and in particular in the teachings, we say that a human being is composed of body, speech, and mind. This is our condition. Sometimes we have illnesses related to the physical level alone: in that case it is easier to cure, to overcome, the problem. But many times not only the physical level but also our energy level is involved. In this case it is a little more difficult, we need deeper knowledge.

But our existence is much more than just the physical level: the mind is even more significant for us. So medicine must correspond with all three existences of human beings; the physical level alone is not sufficient. Only then is medicine complete. In our society, in our attitude, we always tend to separate things. We feel that medicine has to do only with doctors. If we hear of some kind of teaching related to the human condition we do not think it is particularly important. For example, we say: "Oh, this is religion, it is not medicine!" We must understand that our existence is made up of body, speech, and mind. Mind is the deepest and most complicated.

Mental disturbances are much more difficult to treat than any kind of illness at a physical level. This is why in the Buddhist tradition one of the Buddha's names is Great Doctor, Great Physician. Buddha's teaching is that our existence of body and speech or energy level is dependent on our mind, that the mind dominates all. Today, when we say that Buddhism is a kind of religion, then we have the limitation of different religions. Buddha did not teach that way. Buddha taught, made us understand, how our situation is. This is also relevant for medicine. For example, the characteristic of Tibetan medicine is not only scientific like the medicine that developed in modern society. Many teachers, like the Buddha and bodhisattvas, have a kind of knowledge that depends not only on our eyes, ears, and organs of senses. They have a capacity of wisdom going beyond that. Just like Buddha.

In Tibetan medicine we also have the Buddha of Medicine. This means that many aspects of Tibetan medical knowledge originally developed from teachings, from understanding. Tibetan medicine did not actually originate from someone cutting the body open or analytically developing that knowledge. But today, when we cut open bodies and check and study and analyze scientifically, the results correspond exactly with the way enlightened beings taught and explained. So it is crucial for us to know the real condition of human beings and the meaning of medicine without just focusing on the material aspect. We need to pay more attention to the energy level, not just the material level. The energy level is more complicated than the physical level.

For example, if someone is approaching, you look, recognize, and say: "Oh, George is coming!" Why? Because you know what George looks like. This is the physical level. We can understand easily: the physical level is something we can touch, we can see. If George would no longer have a body, only energy, and if his energy were coming here, we could not see him. To be able to see the energy level you need the capacity of clarity, you cannot see it in an ordinary way. We are living in an ordinary way: we have five senses based on five sense organs and we are completely dependent on them. If we close our eyes we cannot see anything. The same is true of the other organs. We are completely dependent on them.

Developing our knowledge, understanding, means to go beyond those five senses. On some figures of deities you can see a third eye. There is a book by Lobsang Rampa that many Westerners may have read. He said Tibetans open the third eye with an operation. That is not true, no one does an operation for the third eye. The third eye is a symbol. We have two eyes that face outward, because we live in dualistic vision. If we want to see something, we open our eyes and see the object: then we have that contact, we can understand. This is also true for hearing, smelling, for all our senses. So everything is perceived in a dualistic way. This is our condition. So, for example, if there is some manifestation of enlightened beings or some kind of beings that are not ordinary, we cannot see them, we cannot understand what is happening. The third eye is a symbol for having developed that capacity. This just helps you to understand how is the situation of our existence of body and speech.

Our mind is much more complicated. Many people say: "I have some problems, something is wrong, I want to go to a doctor." They go to a doctor, they are checked in the hospital and the doctor says there is no problem. Then they go home. But in a real sense, just because the doctor says there is no problem it does not mean the person has become healthy. The problem still exists. Why? Because that illness is something more related to the energy level. In Tibetan medicine, for example, we learn that one of the first things to check is whether a condition is *dönchen* and *dönmed*. *Dönchen* means connected with negative provocations. *Dönmed* means there is no problem of this type; it is more on a physical level. Even if the disorder has to do with our energy level, it is not the same as *dönchen* and there is a way to coordinate the energy.

These days in the West, many people are interested in learning and doing practices like yoga. Why is it beneficial? Because it coordinates our energy when there is some kind of disorder. In general, we live in a dualistic way and apply many things that sometimes create negativities and do not correspond with our condition. Then we disorder our energy or sometimes some functions of the five elements become damaged. And then we become passive, because we do not have sufficient protective energy. Many people say: "I have so many problems. I am doing my best, but everything goes wrong!" I am sure most of you have had this kind of experience. Sometimes even without much effort, whatever you do goes fantastically. Why? Because when there is no disorder or problem with your energy, your energy functions perfectly. At that moment we might say: "This is a moment of fortune, I am very fortunate!" We jump on the idea of fortune, but fortune and misfortune do not really exist. The main thing is our condition: if the function of our energy is perfect everything goes well.

For example, when we follow a spiritual path we might decide to do a practice for long life. What does long life mean? It does not mean just live a little longer, it means a long life with good health, with prosperity, with coordinated energy, so that everything goes well. So we need to know that the energy level is one of the most important aspects of our existence.

I remember many years ago once I went to some places in Italy to speak about Tibetan medicine. I explained that in Tibetan medicine we also use mantras. Many people did not know what a mantra is. Mantras are words that have a specific potentiality and we can produce that function. Then they asked how mantras work. Originally, any mantra must have been pronounced by someone who empowered [the sound] to have that kind of function. An ordinary person could not do that. Only someone having that specific realization and potentiality could put that transmission in a sound. We need to receive that sound, this is called transmission of the *lung*. It is not an explanation of how we do a practice, that is called instruction. *Lung* means we are simply listening to this sound, because the potentiality is in the sound.

When we study Tibetan medicine there are also many mantras. Therapy and mantras go together. They work for many different kind of illnesses and can help us overcome specific problems. But we cannot expect that all we need to do is recite a mantra and it cures every illness. Some people have this idea, but it does not work that way. If you use a mantra, its potentiality helps increase the effect of the medicine, of the therapy you are doing. And mantra is sound; sound is connected with our energy. When we speak of the three existences of the individual in Tibetan we say *lü*, *ngag*, and *yi*. *Ngag* means voice, or sometimes we say speech. The voice or speech is related with our breathing. Our breathing is our life. When we are inhaling and exhaling, inhaling and exhaling continuously, we have the continuation of life. If we stop there is no life. But this breathing is connected with our vital energy. The vital energy is the most important energy for the individual condition. When we discover that our energy is disordered, what can we do to coordinate and strengthen it? We should work with the vital energy. Vital energy is connected with breathing. You know very well how it works, for example in yoga or specifically Yantra Yoga. Working with a combination of sound, visualization, and so on, we can coordinate our energy. If our energy is damaged or weak we can strengthen it. This is because it is connected with breathing and breathing is connected with the vital energy.

In very profound, ancient teachings, sound is explained as the origin of all manifestations. Today scientists are discovering the same thing and they are starting to talk about this. From emptiness, how do all manifestations, all qualifications, manifest? Through sound. The sound we produce with our breath when we are talking or communicating something is called speech or voice. So that is connected with vital energy, for that reason in Tibetan the second of the three existences is called voice.

The third is mind. Body, speech, and mind are the three existences we all have. If these three are in perfect condition there are no problems, we are living well. Tibetan medicine is based on three humors (*lung*, *tripa*, and *peken*), and Ayurveda follows a similar principle. Many people jump to the conclusion that *lung*, *tripa*, and *peken* are illnesses. But they are not illnesses, they are three energies existing in an individual's condition. If *lung*, *tripa*, and *peken* are perfect we live in a perfect state. If they are not working well and there is some disorder we have illness. Only then we can speak of disorders of *lung*, disorders of *tripa*, or disorders of *peken*.

Our condition also consists of five elements; it is the same for all of us from the beginning of our life. When they are harmonized everything is perfect, there are no problems. This is something important for people to understand. Sometimes when there are problems a person becomes upset, saying: "I can't help it, everything is going wrong." In this case, instead of being upset you must understand. The reason is that your energy level is disordered, you need to coordinate it. How do you coordinate? There are many ways.

For example, in Tibetan medicine we speak of *se*, *jöd*, *man*, and *ched*; these are four principles. *Se* means diet, different kinds of diet. *Jöd* means attitude, how we are living, what we doing. *Man* means medicine, different kinds of medicine for specific illnesses. *Ched* refers to different kinds of therapies, such as moxibustion, massage, and so on. In Tibetan medicine we have twenty-one different kinds of therapies, not just moxibustion or two or three others. We can use these as methods to coordinate and harmonize. This kind of coordination can focus specifically on the physical level or the energy level or the mental level. You can also combine different therapies.

For example, yoga can help us coordinate disorders of our energy, strengthen our energy and so on. We do it through breathing, positions, and movements. And other practices consist of three aspects as well: mantra, mudra, and visualization. This is because we have body, speech, and mind, so those three aspects correspond. Mudra means gestures we present with our hands or body. They are a way to communicate with enlightened beings and have very precise functions. Mantras, as I said earlier, are words that have a potentiality. Visualization involves working with our mind. When we combine together mantra, mudra, and visualization, of course we can have the function of the practice we are doing. When we speak of practice, some people think, "Oh, this is religion, this is spirituality" and do not accept. This is not understanding the real sense of the teaching. It is better not to limit ourselves that way. If there is something useful for overcoming problems we should use it. There is no need for any kind of limitation.

So as I mentioned earlier, in Tibetan medicine we first distinguish between *dönchen* and *dönmed*. Dönchen means having negative provocations. For example, today we have illnesses like cancer, AIDS, and paralysis. These kinds of illnesses cannot be cured with medicine alone; it is not so easy. This is because they are also related to negative provocations. Negative provocations can be related with our condition. For instance, maybe we did something wrong or we ate something wrong, and we can receive this kind of negativities. But many negativities come from creating problems with other sentient beings. This can easily happen, though in general we do not believe very much. If someone says there is a spirit, for example, many people do not believe it. And if we ask them why they do not believe they answer: "Because I never saw this kind of beings." They think this is logical, but it is not. A great Tibetan scholar of the Sakyapa tradition, Sakya Pandita, said: "Just because you do not see something does not mean it does not exist." For example, we cannot see behind this wall, but we cannot say that something behind it does not exist. Sometimes it is related to time, sometimes to space; we do not know. If you do not believe, just look at the sky one night, a clear night, and see how many stars there are. You know very well that stars – just like constellations and solar systems – are infinite. And how can we believe that all these kinds of dimensions are empty? Many kinds of sentient beings exist, big and small. Also many tiny sentient beings exist on our earth that we cannot see, for example. And in particular we can provoke them without knowing it because we are ignorant that they exist. In Tibet when you cut down trees or cut into mountains, and so on, we say you can create problems with the local guardians who consequently direct negativities at us. When we receive that kind of negativity it is not so easy to overcome. It can affect the person, the family, even generations. And then we have to pay. When our condition becomes weaker we are paying. This is the result of negative provocations. So it is important to first determine, when there is an illness, whether or not there is what we call *dönchen*. If there is, and if you know a teacher who can help with that, you can recommend the person to seek advice.

Let me give you an example from my experience. Once I went to the United States, to a Kagyüpa dharma center in Boston. They had asked me to come and give a talk there. Just before the talk a very elegant gentleman came and asked to speak with me. I thought he wanted to know something about Tibetan culture and knowledge, so I said: "I am supposed to give a talk now. We can speak when I finish." He said OK. Then I went inside and started to give the talk. The hall had large windows, we could see outside, there was a kind of big garden. This gentleman was walking up and down, waiting for me. I thought he would come inside to listen to my talk, but he did not. Then I thought: "Strange! Then what does he want to talk to me about?" When I finished and went to my room he arrived and said, "I heard you are not only a Tibetan teacher, but also a Tibetan physician. I have some problems and I want to have some advice." I asked what kind of problem he had and when he explained I understood very clearly that he was starting to develop the illness of paralysis. So I told him he should treat the problem not only with medicine, but also do a practice for coordinating the function of his energy otherwise even medicine and therapies would not work. "What should I do?" he asked. "You should do Vajrapani practice," I said. "Do you know what Vajrapani is?" "No." "But are you generally doing some practices or following a teaching?" "Yes, I have been following a teacher for seven years and I am doing practice." Then I said: "Very good, ask your teacher to give you the transmission of Vajrapani. Try to do this practice and also take medicine, then the therapy will work. It is very important that you do that." He said OK and that was it.

The next year I went to the same place to give a talk and he came back again. His condition was a little worse, not like before. I asked him if he did Vajrapani practice. "No, not yet," he replied. "Why? Didn't you ask your teacher?" "Yes, I did, but he said I should first finish the preliminary practices and I could not finish the prostrations because in my condition it is very difficult." So he had not received the practice of Vajrapani. I said it was very important, but he did not ask me to give him Vajrapani, otherwise I could have helped. He was a little limited that way. But at least that time he came to listen to my talk. When I saw that he was present I also explained particularly to make him understand. When the talk was finished he went away.

Then I did not see that man for three or four years. When I went to Tsegyalgar, the Dzogchen Community base in Massachusetts, and we started our retreat, one day he arrived with a dog. He had become blind. He could not walk very well. Then finally he was interested to receive Vajrapani. But it was too late. I gave him Vajrapani, also he followed my teaching retreat. After one or two years when I returned there I asked people where this gentleman was, what had happened to him. He had passed away. That is an example. Our life is very short. We are living in circumstances and there are so many negativities. We need to coordinate our energy, strengthen our energy. This is also part of medicine. So we should not consider that medicine is only something we take in our mouth. We should understand our existence of body, speech, and mind.

I will not be able to come to the roundtable this evening as scheduled in the program. So if someone has some questions I could answer now. In any case it is very good that many Western and Eastern doctors are present here: we really need to open up and promote more collaboration. Tibetan medicine is very valuable, but it is not as diffused as others like Ayurveda and Chinese medicine. This is because Tibetan medicine as well as Tibetan culture, knowledge, and spiritual path, remained isolated for centuries and centuries. Even though it was isolated, in ancient times in Tibet there were many powerful kings who invited teachers from India, from China, from different places. They also invited many Tibetan doctors who were experts in Tibetan medicine and Tibetan astrology, so the knowledge of medicine and other sciences is highly developed in Tibet. But even though it is quite advanced, it is not particularly well known. So it is especially important today, in this world, that people who are interested in medicine and other sciences try to learn and integrate not only the knowledge of medicine but any other aspects of Tibetan culture as well. There are many valuable things and no one knows how long they will still exist. The Tibetan situation is weak, because Tibetan culture and knowledge are related to Tibetans and Tibetans are slowly slowly disappearing. Maybe you do not know it, but Tibetans have exceptionally rich spiritual knowledge, books, language, writings, and so on, with centuries of history. But today there is no use for these things, new generations always have to study Chinese. They have knowledge of Chinese culture but the knowledge of Tibetan culture and language is very weak, because they have no possibility to study. So if we go on this way for one or two generations Tibetans will disappear. Knowing that, we must take care not to lose this heritage. It is valuable and we must save it and integrate it in this world. I think this is something very important.

Q: I would like to ask what would be the ideal result of this symposium, what do you hope it will contribute to Tibetan medicine?

A: I think it is something like opening a door. I couldn't say what specific success our meeting might have, but it is very important we are meeting, that doctors, both Western and Tibetan, can exchange a little and open this door. We are living in time that passes day after day, month after month, we know there is something to do and we can develop.

Q: A commitment from all of us, perhaps?

A: Certainly. What is most important is that we understand what is the real sense of medicine, be it Western or Eastern. To give an example: if someone is ill what that person really needs is to overcome this problem. Knowing this we should work toward integrating [the various medical systems].

Q: I would like to know if the effectiveness of Tibetan medicine has much to do with the culture of the people and the trust that Tibetans have in it.

A: Tibetans know very well how important Tibetan medicine is and also how important its history is. Most Tibetans know. And they always try to promote and develop that. But you must understand in general the situation of Tibet. We cannot do very much even if we have the idea and desire to, including in the field of Tibetan medicine. This is why I am saying it is very important not only for Tibetans, but also for Westerners and everyone in the world to understand that this is something with great value that we must not lose. We need to learn, develop, and integrate. This is what I think.

Q: According to the approach of Tibetan medicine, what is a mental disorder?

A: Mind is in time and space, mind is limited; we follow after the mind. Most people are dominated by the mind instead of dominating and using their mind. Then we have these kinds of mental problems. When you go a little deeper with your knowledge, ultimately you discover that our existence is not only mind, that there is also the nature of mind, the potentiality of mind. This potentiality and nature of mind is not inside of time and space. If you want to go deeper into this field you should follow the teachings a little, what we are doing in general, then you can understand. Otherwise, if we are living in time and space only, limited to that alone, it is not so easy for ordinary people to understand what we mean when we say should use our mind. Instead they are following the mind, the mind is dominating them. If you observe a little this way maybe you can understand something.

Q: From the point of view of Tibetan medicine, how can the negative influence of the environment, of the surroundings, and so on, influence an individual's mental health?

A: This depends on the individual. If your condition is disordered and there is not sufficient protective energy, you can receive any kind of negativity, collective or not collective. If your energy is perfect, if you know how to coordinate and strengthen it, you will not receive negativities.

(2nd session)

Dr. Phuntsog Wangmo received her advanced degree in 1988 from the Lhasa University School of Traditional Medicine, where she also served a two-year residency after completing her five-year training program (1983-1990). During that time she studied with the *khenpos* Troru Tsenam and Gyaltsen, two of Tibet's foremost doctors who are credited with the revival of Tibetan medicine within the Tibet Autonomous Region. Dr. Phuntsog Wangmo had the exceptional opportunity to receive extensive clinical training under Khenpo Troru Tsenam for four years. Thereafter, she dedicated many years of work as a doctor in Eastern Tibet, where she collaborated and directed the implementation of A.S.I.A., a nonprofit organization founded by Chögyal Namkhai Norbu. Since that time, she has worked on behalf of A.S.I.A. setting up hospitals and training centers in the remote regions of Sichuan Province and Chamdo Prefecture.

From 1996 to present, she has been the A.S.I.A. project coordinator in Tibet for the development of Gamthog Hospital in collaboration with expatriate personnel as well as the overall health coordinator and practitioner of traditional Tibetan medicine supervising health activities throughout the surrounding region of Chamdo Prefecture. Prior to 1996, she was on the faculty of Shang Shung Institute in Italy, giving numerous seminars and conference presentations on Tibetan medicine. Dr. Wangmo is based at the Shang Shung Institute of America, where she is the director of the Institute's Traditional Tibetan Medicine Program.

PRESENTATION

PHUNTSOG WANGMO:
Bridging Eastern and Western Medicine

Good afternoon everybody.

Thank you, Rinpoche.[1] Under your guidance we, the International Shang Shung Institute, have the opportunity to support, preserve, and promote Tibetan culture in the world. All these charitable programs and projects are under your guidance, so today I take this opportunity on behalf of the International Shang Shung Institute to express our deep gratitude to you, Rinpoche, our dear teacher.

I would also like to thank you all, in particular the organizers of this event. I know that organizing this kind of event is not easy nor can it be done overnight; it is a big endeavor. So on behalf of the International Dzogchen Community of which I am a member and on behalf of the International Shang Shung Institute I want to thank the Barcelona Community and everyone who participated, supported, and collaborated to make this event happen. This is what I wanted to say first of all.

Today my topic is how we can bridge Eastern and Western healing arts or medicines. As Rinpoche mentioned before, healing is healing. It does not matter which tradition you are following, it does not matter in which language it is written, it does not matter which title you have. Medicine is medicine and is for the benefit of all sentient beings, belongs

---

1   Respectful Tibetan term used to address a high spiritual master, meaning "Precious One." Here it always refers to Chögyal Namkhai Norbu.

to all sentient beings, and does not belong to any one culture or group or individual.

Since I came to the West I learned there are many different types of healing systems: major ones and minor ones, but all of them have the same two aims or goals: first of all to prevent disease, and if that is not possible try to treat the disease. It does not matter whether you go to the East, to the West, South, or North, all healers or doctors or physicians have these same goals. These are our only goals.

Of course, when we work we all have slightly different systems, based on our culture, based on our system's characteristics: we have slightly different systems, but the goal is the same. As Rinpoche just mentioned, in Tibetan culture and medicine it is very important to understand the body first of all. When I came to the West, to America, ten years ago, I learned there are many types of specialized doctors. Once, I had a physical problem: my lymph nodes were rather swollen. I asked a doctor: "What do you think? I have this lump." She said, "No, that's not my specialty." Then I met another doctor and I thought that was a good opportunity to ask. I did, but she also said, "I am sorry, that's not my specialty." Then I said, "Okay, which kind of doctor are you?" "I am a psychologist." This was how limited my knowledge was since it was practically the first time I heard that there are doctors called psychologists and patients called psychological cases. That does not mean that in Tibetan medicine we do not have an understanding of mental diseases nor does it mean that we Tibetans do not have mental diseases. Of course, we do have plenty of cases.

In Tibetan medicine, as Rinpoche mentioned, body, mind, and speech are integrated, support each other, work together, and then the body functions. The actions of the body have physical, mental, and verbal functions. These are the three functions of the body. If one of them is not working, there is a disability or a handicap or whatever we want to name it. It means we are not functioning healthily. In order that the body may perform properly, these three need to function together. That is why in Tibetan medicine since the beginning we have a very good understanding of the body, mind, and speech, like siblings or a team, working together. For this reason we do not have a specific doctor called a psychologist and also we do not have a specific type of patient that we call mentally diseased. Once a patient comes to the clinic or visits a doctor, we try to see what in the body is not functioning. If the body is not happy, the mind is surely not happy and the energy is also not healthy. That is the way we treat disease.

How does Tibetan medicine understand mental disease? In Tibetan medicine, mind is seen as a king, the body as an assistant or a servant. We know that when we age our joints ache, our knees swell, we are not able to walk. The body is not able to walk, not able to act, and the mind is worse than it was, as it develops more desires, more hatred, and so forth. It is never tired. The mind is always active. The physical body is aging, getting older, but the mind is not getting older; it always remains as active as a teenager. This is something simple we can see. The mind is continuously active; but the assistant, the body, which is composed of matter, ages. Sometimes these two are not collaborating well because the mind is too bossy and the body is sort of tired. This is also a cause of disease. Today Western medicine and scientists also say that if you have too much stress then you are subject to a lot of diseases. Now they also say that one cause for cancer is stress. I do not think that about five or ten years ago this was being said, but today it is. That means that if of the three, body, mind, and speech, one is affected, the rest gradually can become affected too.

All healing systems can work together; each has its own potentials, its own capacities, its own benefits. Western medicine has many great capacities; sometimes it really saves people in a miraculous way. The same is true also for Chinese, Ayurvedic, and Tibetan medicine. In Western medicine, the therapy or treatments sometimes seem a little heavy, whereas Tibetan treatments may seem too light at times. When we work in the clinical field we can often see these kinds of things. An example: if a woman waiting for childbirth has a complicated situation, Tibetan medicine at this moment cannot do very much. Western medicine instead does miracles and saves both lives. Also it relieves the suffering, making it last shorter, although this sometimes creates some other problems.

Therefore one of our goals for this medicine conference on Integrative Healing is to try to have us all sit together to discuss what we can do in the future and also to see as individuals what we are doing now. We think this is also important to collaborate on in the future.

As we said before, in Tibetan medicine we have an understanding of diseases at a coarse material level, at a more subtle energy level, and at a still more subtle energy level. When we look at mental disease cases, we can *see* that patients manifest anomalous symptoms also on a physical level. For example, their skin color is pale and they talk either too much or too little. And not only on the physical level, but also on an energy level, we can perceive that something is not working: as soon as the mentally affected person comes near we can *feel* that something is not right, that his energy is disordered. But if we start the treatment on only one level and the patient's state of health does not respond then we need to treat both parts, the physical body and the mind. How do we do this in Tibetan medicine? How do we work in these cases?

Since the beginning we must understand that our body is composed of five elements: earth, water, fire, air, and space. As long as these five elements are working as a team our body is functioning and the five elements are supporting each other and collaborating together. As long as they are balanced the body functions well. For example, earth is heavy, so it acts like a frame. Water is to give lubrication or fluidity. Fire has the nature of everything that acts, moves, matures, regenerates. Air moves, especially like energy circulating. And space gives all other elements the chance to develop. This is the basis, like the fundament of all five elements. As long as they are balanced we are healthy. But sometimes these five elements become unbalanced. In what way does the imbalance manifest? Three things can happen according to Tibetan medicine. There can be an excess, there can be a deficiency, or there can be a disturbance. For example, sleep is good and important, it regenerates energy. But if you sleep too much then we say it is not good and we need treatment. If you do not sleep, that is also not good and again we need treatment.

So too much sleep means an excess, too little is a deficiency. If more complex and confusing symptoms linked to sleep occur it means you are suffering a disturbance. These three outcomes exist when we are sick and having a bad time. In that case what is happening? The five elements are unbalanced. There is nothing more than these three cases: everything comes under these three categories.

How do we treat excess, deficiency, and disturbance? How can we create balance? As Rinpoche has mentioned before, there are four methods of treatment: diet, behavior, medicine, and external therapies. In Tibetan medicine, depression is treated on a case-by-case basis. Even if you have the same problem as someone else, the medicine you get is slightly different. Why? We look at the place where you are living, your environment, your age, your basic personality, your constitution, and your primary problems, all of those things, plus in which season you are having these problems. All this information is put together: then we decide what kind of treatment you should get. Why? Because environment, season, and so on are the outer elements, and in Tibetan medicine we have a very good understanding of how the outer elements affect the inner elements, of how outer and inner elements are related.

When we look at a season we can see with our own eyes how things change outwardly. Spring comes, leaves bloom; summer comes, all flowers bloom; autumn comes, all the seeds are mature; winter comes, everything goes back to being as if frozen, or resting. We can see outside the four seasons changing, but we cannot see how our body's *inner* condition is changing: our eyes are not designed to be able to see momentary changes and especially not in ourselves. It is not only our body we cannot see, but sometimes also we cannot see our negativity. We are able and expert at blaming others but it is difficult for us to see what we are doing. If we could do so easily, probably there would be less fighting and discussions. One of the reasons why we are not able to see much of what we are doing is because our eyes are pointed outward. We are very good at seeing what other people are doing. Thus we are able to see the outer nature but we are not able to see the inner nature. When one is changing over time, the other is also changing. That is why for Tibetan medicine it is important not only to know your nature and your condition, but your whole environment. When we look at the climate, and the characteristics of the land – humid or desert-like and so forth – different diseases also present themselves. When living in a humid place more people have arthritis. Senior or aged people who have pain in the joints or elsewhere like to go to warm places. Why? Because the antidote for humidity is the desert. So the environment is also important: to understand where the person is living, in which season you have problems, what your personal constitution is. All this information is the basis for the diagnosis.

And then one arrives at the personal, individual history: what is your lifestyle? A lot of diseases and problems are also connected to one's lifestyle. That is quite obvious. If we have a peaceful job, boss, or colleagues, we are more healthy. Having a difficult boss or work environment puts us under tremendous stress, as much or more than the actual job we do. We also look at what you eat, what kind of diet you follow. We put all this information together to create the second basis for diagnosis.

Finally, we have thirty-eight different methods of diagnosis included in three systems: checking the pulse, looking at the eyes and especially at urine samples, and, most important, questioning the patient. We use all three of these sources of information in our diagnostic system. Then we finalize the diagnosis of the pathology. Once we have decided on the pathology and what problems you have, it is classified under its Tibetan medicine category. Mental diseases in Tibetan medicine come under five different chapters. On the topic of anxiety alone, there are many different types, not just one or two. Now we decide which category your anxiety belongs to, which your depression falls into, and which your hallucinations belong to. Based on that, we decide what kind of treatment you need.

Once we apply the treatment, we need to treat the physical, mental, and energy bodies, so for the problems of these three we also need medicines at three different levels: physical, energy, and also mental level medicines. More simply we say physical or material medicine and energy level medicine. Thus they fall into two categories: visible and invisible. Visible medicine is when we change the diet, change the lifestyle, if necessary introducing some supplements as well, all of which are more on the material level.

Another treatment, similar to practice, is that of changing your mental attitude. So you need to understand that your mental capacity or functions are not something that works with material medicine. That is, you need to know what the mind is, how to manage it. As Rinpoche said before, for these kinds of things you need to understand or study what is more like the Buddhist teachings. Studying Buddhist teachings does not require you to be a Buddhist, or join a religion, or political party. Most of what Buddhism explains is more like which kind of social conduct you should have. It explains how you can be peaceful, enjoy being human, and appreciate a meaningful life and how you can control or manage your emotions. This kind of understanding of the mind is more related to the teachings. You need to understand and learn this through the medium of language.

Another approach is yoga. Yoga involves coordinating physical movement and breathing.

Dementia in the understanding of Tibetan medicine is related to *lung*, *tripa*, and *peken* [the three humors in our body] and to the five elements. For example, earth and water elements are located in the upper part of the body but they function in the lower part of the body because they are heavy elements. As water from the mountain goes down to the valley, the nature of that which is heavy is to go down. If there is too much heavy nature present then we have physical symptoms of heaviness, losing memory, depression and so on. If the condition gets worse what happens is that in the brain the earth and water elements collapse. When we look with a Western medicine tool such as X-rays, we can see that the brain of those who suffer this condition has hole-like lesions. But Tibetan medicine explains that the earth-water elements are too heavy, in excess, and are unable to be stationary and thus fall down.

What do we need to do to prevent that or to treat the earth and water elements when they are too heavy? The antidote of heaviness is lightness. The antidote of liquidity is dryness. So we do physical exercise and when we do the body develops heat and wind. So that is of help. Second, we coordinate the breathing. The nature of breathing is light and rough. We coordinate the breathing through many types of exercises. I know that several yoga teachers are in this audience. Today I am not aiming to promote our yoga: I just want to explain what yoga is. Any kind of yoga is certainly good. What is our Yantra Yoga? In Yantra Yoga there are three things we need to do: move the physical body; coordinate your intention, your mind; and meanwhile coordinate your breathing. Through these three, the body moves and coordinates the breathing to accumulate heat – light, roughness – to help to reduce the sticky, heavy, cool, wet nature of the earth-water elements. That is the way to help.

Western medicine has a great way of working but sometimes I feel – I may be wrong, in that case I apologize – that it is a bit like a very smart, very active, teenager with a lot of energy and will to do that sometimes perceives the body as a machine: cutting something from here, inserting something there, and so forth in a mechanical way at times. And I feel Tibetan medicine is a bit like a well-experienced, grounded elder, who also sees clearly and knows. Can you imagine a family where teenage boys and girls are living with their grandparents? And both are healthy, no? I feel this is similar. If practitioners of Eastern medicine, a very rich and grounded knowledge, and of Western medicine, a very new, developing and dynamic knowledge, try to work together and combine their skills, each with open minds, it can be very effective. Our priority needs to be that we as healers, or doctors (the term you want to use to call us is unimportant, we are all simply people who work in the medical field since our aim and goal is to help sentient beings) take responsibility and try to open our minds and conduct research. If we see that one medical system lacks the ability to completely resolve an issue, we try to use other approaches. For example, in defining pathology Western medicine does not find the environment so important; nor lifestyle; nor most feelings. Importance is attributed only to symptoms.

In Tibetan medicine symptoms are not so relevant. Of course it is important to understand what is wrong. Symptoms are like a manifestation, a bit akin to putting on makeup or not, it is of little importance. Symptoms are like one day I am dressed in bright colors, one day I am dressed in very dark clothes, but it still is the same me. So in Tibetan medicine, symptoms are not very important: the main thing is to understand the root of the disease. To do so we need all this information to identify precisely what is wrong, what are the excesses, deficiencies, and disturbances. For example, why is there an excess? Suppose there is an excess, but why that kind of excess? Say you live in a desert, a windy place. It is summer, the rainy season or there is a lot of wind. Your age is advanced. Furthermore your lifestyle is that normally you eat light and dry food, mainly food like lentils, not meat or dairy products. Plus you have a stressful job. All these things for us are important bits of information to understand what is wrong, to reveal what the pathology is. Once we have found out these things, physically we can take appropriate medicine, but mentally, which is more important still, as I have said before, one can meditate and learn how the mind works and how to deal with it. Many Buddhist teachings explain trying to understand impermanence. Learning about impermanence is a great help to reduce hatred, jealousy, and also to learn how important it is to show other people respect and loving kindness and harmonize one's relations with them. All of these are usually called Buddhadharma, but, in fact, it is social conduct. To learn this is also part of the treatment. Then we have many other kinds of treatment.

It would be good to see how a bridge between these two medicines can be built. In Western medicine there may be some information missing relating to how to do a thorough diagnosis. It would be good to understand why someone is not happy or in other words, to understand the cause or the root of the symptom. Once the root of the symptom is understood maybe it would be helpful to take Western medicine, and also to do some yoga or to coordinate one's breathing or to do some external therapy. There are many ways these two medicines can be bridged.

Before I came to the West I had been working for many years in remote areas in Eastern Tibet. I did not have painkillers to reduce pain. I did not have anti-depression medication either. All patients' problems needed to be resolved using natural medicine and remedies, and these worked very well, not only for me, but for centuries and centuries for Tibetans receiving these kinds of treatments. The history of Tibetan medicine spans five thousand years. Since in the Himalayan plateau there were human beings, to this day we have been living with these kinds of natural remedies. Tibetan medicine in Tibet is not something new; it has been used since many thousands of years by the Tibetan forefathers. With these techniques we managed to cope with all our issues and we should be able to do the same if we use them in modern society. Today we have a lot of healing systems but we also have a lot of problems, a lot of diseases. If we were able to use these kinds of simple techniques, there would be less side effects with less expense. When we study Tibetan medicine it is said to have eleven advantages, but since I came to the West I have seen more than eleven. One is it is also very easy to apply, gives great benefit, and is inexpensive. Can you imagine how much it costs a year to keep a mentally ill person medicated with anti-depression pills?

One time I had to buy psychiatric drugs for a friend who had a problem – today I do not have time to tell the whole story. Anyway we in the Tibetan community had to buy medicine for him. One pill cost twenty-one US dollars. Ideally he needed to take that medicine for the rest of his life. So we in the Tibetan community somehow had to come up with that money. In the meantime I was going to Venezuela. Then the Tibetan community told me that they had heard that in Venezuela everything costs less than in the US and asked me to try to buy the medicine there. In Venezuela I went to different pharmacies trying to find that medicine: one pharmacy sold it for eleven dollars. True, it cost less than in the US, but it was still expensive. Then we went back to the doctor and said we could not afford this medicine for the rest of his life and that it was too costly for us. Moreover it did not sound like this medicine was mild and we asked what kind of side effects my friend might expect. He gave us three pages full of all the possible side effects: hair loss, damaged teeth, and many more, none of them good. When looking at these three pages – we read everything as if it were homework – we found there was nothing good there. What was the benefit in taking it? That for twenty-four hours it kept the patient under control, that was its function. We tried to take him wherever we went, parties and so on, because he looked so depressed, but no matter where we would go he was always just sitting in a corner. Whatever we did for him was useless, nothing interested him. So we failed.

This is an example. To keep one person on an anti-depression treatment is very expensive. The money for that needs to be found by the family, community, society, and onward back to the country or nation. If one of these people were to be able to manage by using simple, natural medicine and techniques – like Yantra Yoga, breathing, exercising and so forth – it would be more pleasant to receive the therapy, have no side effects, and would also have a low cost. I think this would be very good. We can see what its value would be, and what benefit it would bring.

In Tibet there is a major Western hospital that hosts a Tibetan medicine department and in a major Tibetan medicine hospital we have a small Western medicine department. Why? In Western medicine, for example, surgery is performed. I studied orthopedic surgery. After surgery, patients need to recover, so in Tibet they take Tibetan medicine. For any kind of disease after receiving certain Western treatments they take Tibetan medicine. Sometimes when the Tibetan diagnosis does not quickly return an answer we perform a Western diagnosis and then prescribe the Tibetan treatment. Also now in the US, for example, my friend, doctor Gesan, works in the oncology department. What do they do there, how are they organized? Twice a month, patients are sent to him from the oncology department and he checks them. The doctors send him patients who are weakening or are receiving chemotherapy or whose liver or spleen are not working. Then they check on the basis of his Tibetan diagnosis. He advises the patients on lifestyle aspects, such as which kind of diet they should follow, what lifestyle habits are more effective and therapeutic, and, if they need, which kind of supplements, or which kind of external therapy like massage, oil treatment, moxibustion, or yoga breathing they could benefit from. These all work together. This would also be, I think, a good way to link the two medical approaches. Now in the US, in the West, there are numerous hospitals, many oncology departments starting to use massage and these kinds of therapies. I think this would be a good point where we can join approaches.

Thank you for listening.

(3rd session)

Dr. Paolo Roberti di Sarsina holds a degree in medicine and surgery and is a specialist in psychiatry. A researcher and prolific author of medical articles, he teaches at various Italian universities and is a prestigious lecturer.

He has run the mental illness units of various healthcare centers in Italy for many years and currently plays a fundamental role in Italian nonconventional medicine. He is the only Italian researcher who advises the World Health Organization under the WHO Traditional Medicine Strategy 2014-2023.

He is an expert in psychiatry and nonconventional medicine for the National Health Council of the Italian Health Ministry; coordinator of the master's degree program for "Health, Traditional and Nonconventional Medicine Systems" at the University of Milan-Bicocca (Italy); and founder and president of the Associazione per la Medicina Centrata sulla Persona ONLUS, Bologna (Italy). His presentation bears the title: *Traditional and Nonconventional Medicine: a Multi-Contextual Approach.*[2]

---

2   We regret that for technical reasons it was not possible to include Dr. Roberti di Sarsina's presentation in this publication.

(4th session)

Dr. Inma Nogués Orpí holds a degree in medicine and surgery from the University of Barcelona, specializing in family medicine. She also holds a master's degree in traditional medicine from the Bosch I Gimpera Foundation of the University of Barcelona and a diploma in homoeopathy. She is author of *De lo físico a lo sutil* (From the Physical to the Subtle), published by Elsiguentepaso, and coauthor of *Medicina natural basada en la evidencia* (Natural Medicine Based on Evidence).

Dr. Orpí has been involved as a teacher in introductory courses to traditional medicine in the field of primary healthcare. She is a professor for the master's degree in traditional medicine and the master's degree in neural therapy at the Official School of Doctors of Barcelona (COMB) and the San Juan de Dios University School.

She currently practices family medicine at a social security clinic in Espulgues (Barcelona). She is president of the nonprofit association Merry Human Life Society (Merrylife) – a platform for the development and expansion of conscience and integrative medicine center – and coordinator of the Health Group of the National Values Plan of Catalonia (Plan Nacional de Valores) being implemented by the regional government of Catalonia through the Regional Social Welfare Council.

PRESENTATION

IMMA NOGUÉS
The Approach to Healthcare within the National Values Plan of Catalonia

I really wanted to be here. For me it is very important and it is an honor to be with all of you at this symposium. We are gathering the results of this National Values Plan. Pepa Ninou wanted to present it, but unfortunately she cannot be here, so I am going to present this plan because we hope it is a seed that will generate fruit. We think this is an incredible opportunity. Five years ago when we started it was a utopia, an idea, a project. Today, the project already has a bit more substance and right now 500 people are working on it. Sixteen groups have been created in various sectors of society, including economy, education, organizations, environment, politics, and health. A lot of sectors are involved in this plan.

We all work in society and are part of it. We have joined forces to work for a better future. The project is called the Values Plan. It is under the auspices of the government but it has not been formally presented yet. We still need to refine it a bit more so for now it is just one small seed; however in the next few months it will be presented to the government. So we are actually advancing more quickly than we thought. I am the coordinator of the National Values Plan for the health sector and I am very aware that the change we are witnessing at this time is radical. This is why the government has given us the opportunity to form a plan. We think this is something extraordinary. A similar project was pursued in Iceland and we had the opportunity to see what they experienced there. They had a very broad group with members from every level of society thinking about how they want their country to be. We are also a group of people here in Catalonia trying to devise a plan that involves many, many sectors. I am going to talk about the health sector.

I wanted to highlight things that we may already know but that I think are really important. For example, the Universal Declaration of Human Rights, in article 25, says that every person has the right to an adequate standard of living, which is important because otherwise there will be repercussions on their health. Poverty, for example, is the main cause of diseases. That is why social justice and solidarity are fundamental values and we need to take them into account, especially now and especially during this crisis because right now we are losing many values. So every person has the right to an adequate standard of living in order to guarantee the health and well-being of themselves and their family, especially with respect to food, clothes, and medical assistance. In Almaty, [Kazakhstan,] the World Health Organization (WHO) confirmed its commitment to health for all as a universal goal. The WHO said that health is a fundamental human right and that one of the main objectives of society is to have the highest possible level of health.

We took this principle into account because we firmly believe in the importance of human rights. And the concept of health involves the whole of society. Health is something that really involves everybody and we need to empower people in this area. One of the things that inspired us in developing this plan is that many of the resources we are using were focused on the resolution of health problems. What we are trying to do is to focus on health even before a disease originates. I think this is essential. Health is a fundamental human right and many sectors contribute to it. According to the WHO, governments have a responsibility for the health of their people and health can only be obtained with good social and health measures. That is why in our plan we took into account only the social aspects, since they are crucial in order to preserve the health of every single human being.

The WHO [policy drafted at Almaty in 1998,] called "Health 21: Health for All in the 21st Century," incorporated contributions of fifty-one countries and led to a number of related resolutions. The contributors said it will affect close to nine hundred million people and that they wanted to collectively stimulate the attainment of health. So we do believe that the social conditions that enable people to be born, to grow, to work, and to grow old are crucial for their health. Social conditions are fundamental because it is social conditions that really bring about changes in order to improve the health and the life of citizens. Another fundamental objective is social and health equity. We cannot have people who cannot have access to health because they have an economic problem; this is not justice. Justice and health are a right for everybody and that is why we thought of developing this Values Plan. First of all we tried to make a diagnosis and in a second phase we developed the programmatic lines that we will be explaining in more detail.

In this diagnosis we saw that the Catalan health system has been really pioneering, and it is also true that technological, diagnostic, and therapeutic progress have contributed to the improvement of the health of the people. Additionally, we noted that many efforts had been made and many resources allocated to the resolution of health problems and that resources had been allocated to the health system itself as well. However, if we had allocated resources earlier, and focused not just on diagnosis and treatment, but also on the *prevention* of diseases, these resources would have been more useful.

We analyzed the main causes of disease and death and we saw that they were related to lifestyle, to social relationships and conditions, and to the environment. So many of these health problems could have prevented if we had more sustainably managed these resources, which ultimately means allocating resources for education and prevention. In our Values Plan we can see that the education of people is very important and we need to give them the instruments to preserve their health *before* they lose it. When we analyzed the factors that most impact on health, we saw that the impact of personal behavior is around 40%; the impact of family and genetic history is 30%; and the impact of the environment and social conditions is 20%; while the impact of medical intervention is 10%. This latter area, however, is where we allocate most of our resources. We need people to have this education and information.

We thought we wanted to have a plan and this plan had a vision and a hope. What was our vision, what was our hope? To have a healthy and vital country is our intention, our biggest dream. We need to find ways to collaborate to have a healthier country inspiring a model that considers human health a fundamental human right and that considers self-knowledge and self-responsibility crucial for its own health. Integrative medicine is very much about the global health of a person, not only at a physical level, and about a medical system that can also be integrative, egalitarian, and supporting. This was the vision, the mission of proposing this plan. The scheme we have developed consists of three programmatic lines that are the synthesis on which our plan is based.

The first programmatic line is that the person should always be at the core, at the center. We call it the three Vs, for a Vital Catalonia, but it could be any country, any people, any society. The emphasis is on vitality. We say *Vida Vivida con Vitalidad* (live life with vitality). We played with the three Vs.

Next are the three Ss: *Solidaria, Sostenible y Saludable*. It means a supportive, sustainable, and healthy country.

Then we have the three Ps: *Pacientes, Professionales, Provedidores* (patients, professionals, providers). The person is at the core. If in all our health politics we had the people at the core, at the center, we would see how everything would change, then we could also realize and carry out different actions.

So the first programmatic line encourages the possibility of self-awareness, of self-management. We want people to be empowered to manage their own lives, to restructure and balance the physical body, which is essential. Seeing that a person is more than a physical body already represents an advancement. We must have this vision of a person as an individual in a global way, in all its different dimensions; it is really clear that self-control and self-awareness lead to a higher level of health. As a consequence, a person can have a better relationship with himself or herself, and also a better relationship with the environment, with the community, with society, and with circumstances of life.

So with this first programmatic line, we are centering and focusing on health. We are experts in diseases. At university we are taught how to cure and how to relieve diseases and illnesses, but we do not teach and we are not experts at all in sciences, in health sciences, and that means we can get avoid looking for solutions before we lose our health. But in fact it is important to focus on the health of people in a proactive way, to have a full and vital life, also based on an integrated society that encourages and promotes this kind of health with a real sense of self-awareness. And it is equally important to have knowledge of the human being. We have to see the human being as a whole. We have to introduce understanding at schools. It is essential if we want to have a more active role.

What we are seeing in this Values Plan is the commitment to encourage an understanding of the relationship between this physical aspect, the physical body, with which of course we are already very familiar, and the environment, an acknowledgement of the importance of external and internal care. We have a lot of medical tools, criteria, like the Hippocratic medical criteria. We need to see medicine as the science of health and integrate it with the care of the internal aspects of the body. This is very important for the work we have to do. Of course we need to acknowledge the central role of lifestyle habits in the balance of health and life. We should introduce this kind of knowledge and science in schools. As Hippocrates already said, nature is healthy. That is something we have to recover and take into account.

And then health relates not only to this physical dimension; we have to go beyond it, we have to give more value to the mental and emotional level, taking into account feelings, how to manage them positively, and teach that in schools. Our internal world is the combination of all these emotions, together with the mental dimension, the world of thoughts and ideas. There we can create the world based on our feelings, based on our thoughts, which is such an important aspect of our constitution.

Then we can manage to become healthier people, taking into account our universities, our medicines, and our schools, and integrating them into this new knowledge. We must take into account the dimension of the person because we are living in an environment, an environment which is a world of relationships, relationships with parents, with your children, with your friends, with your wife or husband. And then there is also the relationship between communities and countries. It is a social world. And solidarity is important. Not thinking only of oneself: we must take into account the rest of the people, to have a healthier society – healthy people in a healthy society – and also to take into account the spiritual dimension of the person. Sometimes we are afraid to include the spiritual part that completes a person. We are afraid to include in our medicine the part that represents the most profound aspect of the person, the part that goes beyond ourselves. It is transcendent because it really gives value to life. Our spiritual aspect is essential and should be integrated.

So what we want to achieve in this programmatic approach is to try to improve the health of people through awareness and a proactive way to live a much fuller and more vital life. That is only possible if you have a fair and integrative society that takes into account this kind of self-awareness and self-knowledge. We can design this new society based on three targets. The first target is the self-knowledge and the pillar of trying to build health and different dimensions. The second target is having the tools and helping people self-manage the various challenges they face, important life changes like losing a loved one, mourning, giving birth. Those are important and vital processes and we need to include them in schools, in the things we teach, so that people can develop tools during their school life. I am a general practitioner and I see so many health problems every day that would not be necessarily have to be cared for at national health institutes if we were able to introduce a different kind of health studies, health teachings, in schools. The third target is to be able to have a really healthy and fair society, that is, living a vital life; you cannot consider that society is really healthy if it is not sensitive and co-responsible for helping and integrating its most vulnerable parts.

We are all vulnerable, and that brings us to the second programmatic line, solidarity within Catalonia, solidarity within a community that is sustainable and fair, a society that is able to see health as something global, something fundamental and universal. That is the general idea. We want to encourage solidarity and that is very important in these times of cost-cutting, of crisis, of financial losses. In times like these we do not have the same possibilities to have access to the national health system. We also have to encourage and promote the co-responsibility of all parts of the health system. This way, from a global and general perspective we can also act locally and bridge the various gaps we have in the health system. We can consider health something that everyone has a right to, that all citizens are part of all systems, not only administration. And we have to include these ideas and this programming in all the parts of society, administration, schools, education, and so on. We know that by reaching all parts of society we can achieve a healthy society. Employment policies, commerce, trade, fair trade, education, universities: these are all areas where we can do many things that can result in benefits for our citizens.

The global crisis we are suffering now demonstrates that there is a need to responsibly use all the resources we have, and that means we have to change the focus of our health systems so that they can be sustainable in the future. This is why we have defined these three targets. The first target is, as we have said, to encourage solidarity and equality and guarantee that people with health problems get the assistance they need, and provide the tools so that people with minor health problems can solve them themselves, and also, of course, help those who are the most vulnerable. The second target is to try to use our resources fairly so that our human and social resources are available for all of us. The third target is to encourage all parts of society to be aware of the active role they have to play in people's health, in the health of society. Not only do employers have to care more, they also have to promote the idea that their employees are the core of the system. We know that many health problems have to do with risk factors and people working in risky environments. For example there are risk factors like smoking, drugs, alcohol, diabetes, high blood pressure, and lack of sports. And we need to remember that poverty and the lack of economic resources are really the main causes of health problems. Again I want to insist that schools, education, and universities are important. Not only because we want to have health experts, but because we want to have experts in people who are healthy as a whole. We need cities and communities where the urban planning takes into account persons, human beings, and where health plays a central role.

In the end, this involvement of the whole of society is what the third and last programmatic line is about, where the person is at the center. The three Ps in Catalonia for People stand for patients, professionals, and providers. We have to inspire a new vision of health in a system that is a paradigm, that is more human, participative, integrating, where we always see the individual, the person, at the core of all fields. We want to encourage the active participation of patients in the entire process of health care, a process respecting the individual, the freedom of the individual, and also making use of the whole system. Professionals must also be more present. We have to promote a confidence and commitment among all professionals, throughout systems and departments, and of course empowering them inside the health system.

Last but not least, we need to take into account that the health system has providers. We must insist that providers put individuals at the core, not only professionals, and we must encourage the patient to participate so that we have a multidimensional vision of the individual and of integrative medicine. Sometimes it is difficult to open the doors, but at this moment we really have the chance to do it and open the vision of integrative medicine. Because there is really only one medicine, consisting of the best of each system and all of them collectively to genuinely help individuals. This vision of helping is so important. We are all participants in building the reality we are living in. In quantum physics anything that we call reality is seen as an active process of building that we are all participating in. We are really in a sea of energy where we can think and feel, and we are part of the reality we are building. The one who is observing is influencing what he is observing, so if we change our consciousness and raise a political and social will and willingness to really build a society that is genuinely fair and a medicine that is closer, where everybody is participating in this vision of health, then we can be able to build something that we are all a part of. We have this responsibility where we are really participants and this vision of integrative medicine that we are developing in this symposium is very important because this medicine already has this vision of the individual in the middle. It is a vision that is not fragmented: it is integrative, it uses mind and body together, it puts more emphasis on life and body and a lot of emphasis on relations between patient and doctor. And the individual is at the core. It is also focused on knowledge and self-knowledge, self-development of this self-awareness and being in charge of yourself. It uses all techniques available and it will be a big step forward. So I think we have to broaden our vision a little bit, maybe change this focus.

To conclude, I would like to say the following: a Tibetan master and doctor said, "Humanity can come out of its state of pain only if we heighten the level of consciousness." This level of consciousness and awareness has to increase so that together we can build a fairer and better world.

Thank you very much.

(5th session)

ROUNDTABLE

Dr. Phuntsog Wangmo, Dr. Paolo Roberti di Sarsina,

Dr. Imma Nogués

Moderator: Ms. Eloisa Álvarez Centeno

Moderator: Now we will have a roundtable where you can address your questions to our guests. Any questions from the floor? Don't be shy. Is somebody breaking the ice?

Audience: A question for Dr. Phuntsog: I understand that traditional medicine may well anticipate and prevent disease during day-to-day life, but how does traditional Tibetan medicine cope with emergencies? If you have an emergency, or an anxiety crisis, or a nerve attack, or something like that, do you think your medicine could also intervene?

Wangmo: Your question is very important, thank you. Many people think Tibetan medicine works only with chronic conditions, that we do not have any system or method to work with acute or emergency cases. So your question allows us to explain a little bit to the audience what we do in these cases. Yes, we do have a traditional system to work with acute or emergency cases, especially for conditions related to the nerves, like a stroke. We do have ways to treat that kind of thing. But honestly sometimes the Western medicine is quicker. So today, since in the major Tibetan medical hospitals – as I explained before

– we have a department for Western medicine, many times people go for that. In case there is something like appendicitis, this kind of acute disease, it seems better to go to the Western hospital. But in the case of diseases related to the nerves, like epilepsy, we are also able to manage in acute situations.

Audience: First of all thank you very much for this presentation, it was very interesting, informative, and Chögyal Namkhai Norbu was certainly an inspiration.

The question I have is: How can we integrate? I live in the USA, I have been there for fifty years and I have seen many changes in psychiatry, for example. Most of them good, I must say. The example you used this morning – of the doctor who works in the oncology department – is not uncommon. Fortunately the USA has been able to introduce more and more the point of view of integrative medicine. So in hospitals it is not uncommon to see a doctor with a special team on complementary medicine, or a holistic doctor, or a Chinese doctor, who does a variety of things including acupuncture. So this is already happening. But it is a country of 330 million people, so we are talking about a big difference between the USA and its culture, which has a variety of different components, and Tibetan culture. How much has Tibetan culture, which you described very well, influenced Tibetan medicine? How can we integrate more and more of this culture and medicine in the USA? Certainly the USA needs those aspects of Tibetan medicine. More and more people are doing yoga, but the interesting thing is that you have to go to class well ahead of time, because if you go at the moment when other people are leaving you are bound to be run over in the parking lot, then it turns into ghost yoga [laughs]. Tibetan culture is so different. So my question is: what can we do to make sure to continue to work toward an integration?

Wangmo: From my point of view there are two ways we can do it. On the one hand there is education, as Dr. Roberti mentioned before, because before we apply things, it is important that you have trust. Trust is one of the powers of healing. If you do not trust, even if I give you something very precious, you think "maybe it works, maybe not," so also the result may not come. I think trust is crucial for every patient because their body is important, their life is precious. If we lose this life or body we do not have any guarantee to get it again. So whatever we receive to guarantee the healing of this precious human life, this body, is very important. The first thing you need to have is that you know what you are doing and you have trust. For this reason there is a need to check if the person who is applying a certain knowledge in your area is qualified or not.

For example, when I arrived in USA in 2001 I did not even know any English at all. Before, I had been in Western countries, in Italy, so I knew a little Italian but no English. My Tibetan colleagues and I had problems communicating and we hesitated to practice Tibetan medicine in America because some people said it was illegal. Then slowly, slowly we improved our communication with people and found out that there is no law in the USA saying Tibetan medicine is legal or illegal. In other words no one had really considered Tibetan medicine from that perspective yet. So that was the issue. Also, in the meantime, we saw that quite a few people in the field were really unqualified. That is why in 2006 we founded an organization we called the American Tibetan Medical Association. Today in this audience most of us are members of that organization, and some of these professors, including Chögyal Namkhai Norbu, are on the advisory committee.

What we are going to do is to establish certain standards for Tibetan medicine. If you hold the title of Tibetan doctor, which kind of qualifications do you have to have? Many people think: "Oh, Tibetan medicine is easy, I just go to listen to a seminar." And then they go to India and spend one week and listen to some seminar. Then they go to Italy and listen to another seminar. Then they go to America and listen to another seminar and then they become doctors of Tibetan medicine and think they can write an article. Tibetan medicine is not like this. Tibetan medicine goes from embryology to death. You need to study anatomy and physiology. In the traditional system it takes two semesters to study just the basic topics. Then, from etiology till pathology, we have 192 chapters to study. When we get to pathology, for example, when we look at the liver diseases, that is one chapter, but it covers seventeen different types of liver diseases. So traditionally we need to study for nine years just to become a basic doctor. In today's society, with the modern techniques or modern methods of study, a bachelor's degree takes five years; a master's four years; and a PhD three years. So we have to study those things one by one, then we become a doctor. *Then* we practice. Tibetan medicine is not something you go and listen to a seminar and then you become a doctor.

This is why the Shang Shung Institute, under Rinpoche's guidance, opened a Tibetan medicine school in the USA in 2005. So far, we graduated three classes: the first batch in 2009, the second in 2011, and the third in 2012. So far we do not have big number of students because for America, alternative medicine is still sort of a dream. Some people feel like dreaming a little, some people still do not dream. But from when I arrived to the present Tibetan medicine has come to the surface and public visibility is improving a lot. As I said before, one of my colleagues is working in the oncology department at Berkley. Another, Dr. Yulha, who is sitting next you, graduated in Tibetan medicine and is now studying Western psychology. Also my sister Yeshe graduated in Tibetan medicine. What we are trying to do is to have our young Tibetan doctors take some Western medicine or classes on other medicines. Then, as we said, we have this school of Tibetan medicine in the US. Many Western doctors also come to the school. We have had Western doctors, Western nurses, acupuncturists, homeopathic doctors, and so on. Right now we have about seven people, from seven countries, with seven different backgrounds.

And now we opened a second school of Tibetan medicine in Russia, in May 2013. It is in its second semester. We have sixty students coming from different parts of Russia and there too we have students from different backgrounds. So I hope Tibetan medicine will become more familiar to people. It is important that first of all you know what Tibetan medicine is, how it works, what its methods are. Once you know its background then you will trust it. I hope our two Tibetan medical schools can do that.

As my colleagues mentioned before, our International Dzogchen Community now has its main seat in Tenerife, in the Canary Islands, Spain. There, too, we will have a big Tibetan medicine program, we want to create an education center and also a practice center. So I am really looking forward to the day when we will all work there and develop the Tibetan medicine center. Our goal is the same. It is not to make money, rather our main goal as healers is to help people who are suffering. I really hope that one day we will work together as a team, all of us healing practitioners or colleagues. We all have the same professional job, we are all entrusted with this responsibility, so it must be that we have a strong karma to work in this field. Really, I am looking forward to seeing you all in Tenerife one day and working on this project. Thank you.

Audience: A question to all of you. How do you explain the great increase in the numbers of psychologically mentally affected patients that we see every single day? From my experience – I am a homeopathic physician here in Barcelona – the number is rising very rapidly. I would love to hear what is your understanding and how we can tackle the problem. Thank you.

Roberti di Sarsina: It would be necessary to have more time to discuss this topic. But anyway we must consider the problem one of the main concerns among social issues. Again I remind you that in the US there are forty million people who do not have any health coverage at all. As our colleagues reminded us, health is a universal ontological right. So in my opinion when you have forty million people without any health coverage it is quite hard to introduce other things when people do not have anything. In Europe, too, we have to face the tremendous burden of side effects due to pharmaceutical products, a lot of problems due to chronic diseases, unemployment, drugs, and social conflicts that are the multiple causes, causes of the enormous growth, for example, of personality disorders, linked to drug use.

Coming back to your question on the enormous growth of mental and social diseases, the huge increase in the comorbidity of personality disorders, drug use, and social inequalities is a time bomb for our so-called post industrialized world. And in my opinion one of the most important duties of our governments must be to reduce social inequalities and unemployment. The problem is also the budget and the huge quantity of people who are seeking work, seeking health care. So we must keep in mind the efforts to promote a salutogenic approach to health. The problem is responsibility, is to strengthen energy, to work together, say no to violence, no to corruption, no to violence against women, boys, children, old people, no to wars, no to pollution. If we have work, human rights, especially starting from minorities, we will have fewer psychiatric illnesses. Thank you.

Nogués: I totally agree with you. From my experience as a general practitioner I see that everyday there is more anxiety, mental disorders, and depression. Why? Because society is sick. We need to see what kind of world we are building. This is really a crisis of values. What kind of world have we built? Maybe we did not know another way, but this crisis, this moment, is a time of tremendous opportunity. This is our time to transform and decide what kind of world we want to build, because the cause of many of these disorders is the way society is being built now. And we are the ones who built this world. So changing our consciousness is going to give us the clarity to know what world we want to build. This is the vision, no?

Wangmo: Thank you. I totally agree with what my two colleagues just said.

As Rinpoche mentioned before, another cause could be that there are diseases arising from provocations in addition to those arising without provocations. I think somehow we have become rough on nature. The way our ancestors took care of nature and the way our generation is taking care of nature is different. I think one cause of the increase of diseases in general, and particularly the mental ones, is that since we have treated nature so badly a lot of these diseases could be considered under the category of diseases caused by provocations. Thank you.

Moderator: To conclude, I want to ask Dr. Imma Nogués whether she would say something about the integration of the different types of medicine in Catalonia, in Spain.

Nogués: One day I presented part of this plan to the president of the college of doctors of Barcelona as well, and he totally agreed with it.

Another time, when I spoke to him about integrative medicine he said, "Yes, this is the way. But the problem is your own colleagues!" And I understand it. I spent six years studying for a medical degree and I remember being in a cafeteria fifteen days before I was to get my degree. One of my colleagues said: "Yes, with homeopathy…" And I said "With what?" "You do not know what homeopathy is? It is another way of healing." I was shocked. I told him, "You are telling me there is another way of healing apart from the one I was taught? And I am going to be a doctor in medicine and surgery in fifteen days!" So it was a shock for me. Many of my colleagues do not know that they are allopathic doctors, and I also did not know it. They do not know there are other medical criteria, such as Ayurvedic medicine and holistic medicine. When they taught me the history of medicine it was never explained to me that other kinds of medicine exist.

So I understand that people might be in shock when you tell them there is another type of medicine. We need an open mind and an open heart to be able to integrate. But I think it is going to really take hold in our society because people are asking for it. Many years ago, we conducted a survey, we asked our patients how many of them had used alternative or complementary medicine. Already at that time 40% of them had turned to some form of complementary medicine, but only 1% of their doctors knew about it. Patients never told their doctors because they were a bit ashamed. As we were not informed that other criteria exist, we did not have that sort of education, on some level there was a sort of rejection of alternative medicine. From my understanding, it seems that traditional medicine has been considered dubious by allopathic medicine. But rather than questioning anything, we simply need to broaden the potentiality of helping. If we look at it from this perspective and if we are able to give this message, doors will open more and more and I think that allopathic doctors will understand it. This is the beginning of a change that will obviously be a slow process. But it will happen. Why? Because society is asking for it, society wants it. I also do some homeopathy and natural medicine and patients ask me to do that. I know there is still rejection because our health structures are the last to change, but I think this is the future, the evolution.

Some years ago I was giving some classes on natural medicine in an outpatient clinic. One of my colleagues told me: "I am listening to you because you are a doctor like me and you work in a practice like me, but if you were not a doctor and if you were not working in a clinic I would not listen to you." I see that little by little many people, on their own, are already promoting [alternative] medicine in the system. Two months ago there was also one-day event on alternative medicine at Terrassa Hospital. Many people were interested and this is something that corresponds with the evolution of our time. This is a medicine of synthesis, a medicine of union, where we can really include the best of everything: this medicine will allow us as humanity to advance and to see the person from a more global perspective. So it is about to happen. Thank you.

Roberti di Sarsina: I believe one of the most important ways to help people is to organize social structures such as foundations or charities. If you like, I propose you share with us and with my colleague and friend Gino Vitiello, who is a distinguished member of my charity in Italy, the idea to set up in Spain, in Catalonia, or wherever, charities whose goal is to promote social empowerment, social awareness. Because the problem is not a matter of homeopathy or acupuncture, but *how* we face the enormous problems of society as a whole. For example, how can we deal with the fact that hundreds of thousands of babies die each year from diarrhea alone. It is abominable. The lack of clean water is just one of the causes. So I propose to share ideas to promote social awareness, social empowerment. Without information nobody can decide properly and wisely for himself or herself. So, in my opinion, we can help by using ethical organizations, such as foundations or charities. Social and ethical organizations, without conflicts of interests, without corruption, are in my opinion among the most powerful ways to help share information and get things done step by step according to the budget or the availability of people who can work. Thank you.

Moderator: With that we are going to conclude today's session. We would like to thank our speakers, we would like to thank Professor Chögyal Namkhai Norbu, and we would like to thank you all for being here. We are look forward to seeing you tomorrow.

Mental Disorders

Saturday, January 11, morning
(1st session)

Moderator: Dr. Eva Juan Linares

Dr. Thubten Phuntsok trained as a doctor in Tibetan traditions and first practiced medicine in his hometown in Derge. He currently works as a professor and researcher at the Tibetan Studies Department of the Beijing Central University for Nationalities in China and is an outstanding scholar of Tibetan medicine and history.

He has written a number of books on a variety of topics. His publications include: *Grammar of Tibetan Language* (1987) Chendug; two volumes on *The History of Tibet* (1994), Chendug; *Elements for the Study of the Physical Condition* (1999), Beijing; *Therapeutic Principles in Tibetan Medicine* (2000), Beijing; *The Relation Between Mind and Body* (2003), Lhasa; and *Elements for the Study of Tibetan Medicine* (2009), Beijing.

He is also director of the Tibetan Medical Institute and president of the Tibetan Association for the Prevention of AIDS (TAPA), which he founded. This is the first nongovernmental organization on the Tibetan plateau dedicated to raising awareness about AIDS and offering medical treatment. He has received numerous national awards for his publications on language, history, religion and medicine, and is a member of the nonprofit organization Machik.

PRESENTATION

THUBTEN PHUNTSOK
Introduction to Mental Disorders
According to Traditional Tibetan Medicine

Good morning friends, I call you friends. I am pleased to have this
opportunity to talk to you about Tibetan medicine. Today my topic is
the idea of global health in traditional Tibetan culture.

As you know, global is a fashionable word these days: we talk about
global warming, global health, and so on. Therefore I too am going to
talk about this, but from the perspective of traditional Tibetan culture
and medicine. Clearly, the more we understand the traditions of Tibet,
the more we will be able to see its connection with the global view. In
Tibet, we have the concept of global health in our daily prayers. Every
day after our prayer or practice we recite this invocation, which is like
a wish, saying:

> May the global ecological system remain healthy
> So that both the harvest and the dharma teachings can flourish,
> So that all auspicious things can be realized,
> And all aspirations can be achieved.

This wish is particularly important today. But it is not a recent idea.
In Tibetan culture, we have always considered global health fundamental. As we can see from this verse in our daily prayers, we were already

wishing the globe to be healthy several hundred years ago. Global health is crucially important: we must keep the health of the environment.

In traditional Tibetan culture, and also in Tibetan medicine, we have always focused on the protection of the environment and we still give it great importance. Also, when we say "global," we are referring not only to the earth but also to all the planets.

The globe according to the Tibetan perspective is considered to be composed of the five elements. The prayer I quoted means that if the globe is healthy then farmers, nomads, our wealth, and the dharma will also be healthy, and our physical body will be healthy too.

Traditionally we have the practice of yoga. The practice of yoga is one of the best ways to live a long life. Actually, the four lines of the prayer include all these aspects and knowledge. The pursuit of health is a common value; of course everybody wants to have a long life with happiness. In Tibetan traditional culture the primary cause for maintaining the health of the physical body is to guarantee the balance of the four or five elements.

What are the elements? I think you know this very well because many of you are students of Namkhai Norbu. Yesterday Rinpoche mentioned what the elements are and what their functions are, so I will just say only a few words about them. The four elements are the fundamental constituents of the universe, the tiny particles of which matter is composed. They are the earth element, the water element, the fire element, the air element. Space is generally considered to be the fifth element, because without space there is no chance for development. The elements are basically the cause of the external world and of the physical body as well.

This idea is quite similar to the periodic table in modern chemistry. It firstly presents how we understand the materials elements. According to the text, we understand the elements with logic. For example, yellow color is earth, blue is water, red is fire, and green is air. Each of the four elements has many properties. For example, the earth element is heavy, stable, smooth, etc. We derive a total of 166 elements from these four. So our elements table is very similar to the periodic table of the elements that is used in chemistry.

The Secondary Causes of Damage to Our Health

According to Tibetan medicine, an imbalance of the elements results in the conditions that damage our health. If we want a healthy physical body we must keep the elements in our body balanced. But of course we have secondary causes to destroy our physical body or to create imbalances. In general we have four secondary causes that can damage our health: atmospheric weather, provocations, diet, and conduct. Let's look at them one by one.

Disease can be caused by atmospheric weather. Normal weather within the various seasons is the cause of a healthy state while weather that is unusual for the season is a cause of disease because it creates an imbalance of the elements of our physical body. In general, the occurrence of unusual weather causes natural catastrophes and is also a result of environmental destruction. Today many people are worried about global warming, which is due to human interventions that destroy the environment. We pay attention to such factors in Tibetan medicine as well.

Provocations are also connected with atmospheric weather because both actually derive from the destruction of the environment. What is a provocation? It means the sudden cause of a problem and includes proximate and remote causes. In Tibetan culture, people usually think they can get damaged directly by nonhuman beings, by the class of ghosts or something like that. The Tibetan term for provocation is *dön (gdon)*, which refers to the eight classes of nonhuman beings. But actually, in the context of medicine, provocation refers on the one hand to any disease that manifests suddenly and may be caused by external agents like pollution or accidents, and on the other hand, in certain cases, it refers to different classes of spirits that are seen as the remote cause of such diseases and problems.

The Proximate Causes

Let us look at the proximate causes. For example, because of unclean circumstances we can have a situation of contamination and consequently problems with blood and wind circulation. For that reason the patient will easily manifest pain, fall unconscious, develop delirium and may end up with depression or schizophrenia. In Tibetan medicine we consider the cause of all these illnesses to be a blockage of wind circulation, or of blood circulation; or maybe the wind could be circulating in a wrong direction, which then causes one to develop hallucinations. Even if objectively something does not exist, the person can see it and then thinks it is a ghost; instead, these visions are caused by wind or blood circulating in the wrong way in the physical body. This is the Tibetan medicine point of view.

Other proximate causes are external accidents such us falling down, being beaten, or being in a car accident.

The Remote Causes

Because people indiscriminately create wastelands, draw water, destroy forests, and pollute the environment, and because of the immoral conduct of people, the eight classes of nonhuman beings get angry and create all kinds of bacteria and viruses. So viruses are the proximate causes of the provocation of diseases, but the eight classes are the remote causes. Of course from the modern point of view, this is more or less considered to be superstition, but this traditional "superstition" also works very well in relation to scientific knowledge. Since we had this point of view, we protected the environment very well in Tibet: even though we lived in high altitudes we had very good forests and extensive grasslands in the past.

Today things are changing. People freely dig the land; water and forests have been destroyed, and natural areas contaminated; people destroy holy places and make pollution by burning unclean stuff – and they kill animals in temples. This means that unfortunately negative human activities are far more developed now than in the past, and because of that the eight classes get angry, as you can see in this copy of a Tibetan medical *thangka*. Consequently they create many diseases, many different kinds of bacteria and viruses, like for example the virus of leprosy. In Tibet we generally distinguish between viruses and bacteria. This is explained in the medical *thangkas*; I did not invent this information; it comes from the ancient literature, from the Four Medical Tantras, which date back four thousand years in history and they explain it very clearly.

Disease is also caused by our diet. Our dietary conduct sometimes becomes harmful for health if we do not use food in an appropriate way: for example, in case of deficient nutrition, or excess of different kinds of elements.

Another cause of disease is our conduct. Unhealthy conduct is deficiency or excess in conduct: for example, deficient exercise of body, speech, or intellect or an excess of physical exercise, speech, and intellectual work. Moral conduct is also included here, but I am not going to explain this, as you for sure already know about it.

The first two of the secondary causes – atmospheric weather and provocations – are influenced by external conditions. To avoid this problem we must collaborate with society: individuals cannot solve this problem by themselves. For example, contagious diseases, epidemics, and infective diseases are the result of the destruction of the balance of the natural conditions. This creates a lot of pollution in the environment. In traditional literature, the different classes of spirits serve as the remote cause for such diseases or problems. You know that today they started to destroy the environment in Tibet like this: they do whatever they like, they dig and mine everywhere, construct bridges, and bring in many electrical services. Now many rivers have disappeared, we cannot find them on the land, they are just underground. So now, even in Tibet, many earthquakes and unusual natural problems happen because of human conduct. According to Tibetan traditional culture the new viruses and diseases, such as AIDS or SARS, a famous disease that developed in Beijing, belong to the class of diseases caused by provocations.

In order to avoid the manifestation of this kind of problem in the future we must make a joint effort, with the whole of society. Once such problems have appeared in society it is hard to get rid of them. Take leprosy, for example: according to historical documents, leprosy appeared in Tibet more than one thousand years ago, the thirteenth king of Tibet suffered from it. But until the 1970s we did not find any cure for it. I think the first doctor who came to China, to Tibet, to cure patients with leprosy came from England around 1977. Even if medicine or science has developed very much today, no single country has yet discovered a cure for AIDS, even though since 1982 many scientists have been doing research on HIV and millions of dollars have been spent on it.

Today many scientists are paying attention to global warming. It is an extremely dangerous situation and a challenge that we must face. According to traditional Tibetan medicine this situation clearly indicates an imbalance of the natural condition. Global warming could potentially produce serious viruses or bacteria like HIV and SARS.

The ancient Tibetan people protected the environment very well because they had to pay attention to the provocations that come from the spirits of the environment. For that reason, before constructing buildings, cemeteries, and so on, first they had to perform rituals to ensure harmony with spirits. People would not dare to destroy nature and its ecosystem. Similarly, they believed that wild animals are the property of the spirits and guardians of the mountains, so taking care of animals as well as they could was part of their basic attitude in life.

So the protection of the environment and of wild animals, as done in the traditional Tibetan culture, proves to be an efficient way to maintain a good relationship with nature and the environment. This belief lasted for thousands of years in Tibet. This is the reason why in the past we had forests, grasslands, but no big roads developed there because we could not destroy the land. So we protected forests very well.

To conclude, people must stop indiscriminately destroying the environment and the rivers, particularly in the East – including in Tibet and China in general. In the West people are starting to protect the environment, but this problem is now also with us, in Tibet.

Thank you very much for listening.

(2nd session)

Dr. María Teresa Herrerías graduated from the Autonomous University of Barcelona (UAB) in 1985 with a degree in medicine and surgery. While studying traditional Chinese medicine at the Setai School in Barcelona (1983-1993), she completed her first specialized studies in homoeopathy in 1989 on a course organized by the Federation of Pharmacists of Barcelona. A few years later, she completed a three-year post-graduate course in Les Heures (1993-1996) and in the years that followed continued studying at various schools in various countries around the world.

She currently works as a homoeopathic health practitioner (homoeopath) and is co-creator of the Sensació Vital de Barcelona study group, as well as a member of WISH (World Institute for Sensation Homoeopathy).

PRESENTATION

TERESA HERRERÍAS
Homeopathic Medicine: Levels of Therapy

Good morning and thank you very much for inviting me here to talk about homeopathy. I was very pleased to listen to the previous presentations starting with Professor Namkhai Norbu, who was saying that disease is not only physical, but also the materialization, we could say, of a disorder that is more profound, an energy disorder. This is a very important principle of homeopathy.

Homeopathy is a medicine, a concept of understanding disease that seems to be very well known because homeopathic remedies are commonly prescribed in pharmacies, with prescriptions based on allopathic concepts of treating causes and symptoms.

I would like to start my presentation by talking about the origin of homeopathy. Homeopathy has an ancestral basis. It started more or less with the father of medicine, Hippocrates, who first presented the basis. It continued with doctors and philosophers of the following centuries, and Hahnemann was the one who really developed it. This will be the first part of my presentation.

Then I will talk about how homeopathy developed and how it related with other philosophers, in particular with Swedenborg, who was more or less a contemporary of Hahnemann. He explained the basis, the foundation, and the philosophical concepts that we can apply perfectly well with homeopathy.

Then I will explain what homeopathy is, and finally I will present a clinical case, what we homeopaths do with a patient. In this context I will explain a concept that has been introduced in this field in recent years, the concept of levels, and at what level we understand mental diseases.

Understanding the Patient from the Perspective of Unicist Classical Homeopathy

Classical homeopathy is unicist, which means we give only one remedy to treat the patient.

Swedenborg, a philosopher and theologian, was born in 1688 in Sweden and had a basic doctrine that he described as the doctrine of utility. Its principles included the theory that nothing exists unless in some way it manifests, that perfection must include its physical manifestation; anything that does not manifest is something incomplete. For example, charity as a thought or concept is positive, but if it does not manifest in charitable acts it does not exist.

Buddhism and Kabala are two streams in which the spirit manifests at a physical level. Swedenborg uses the sun as a metaphor to explain this, saying that light (wisdom) and warmth (love or understanding) both come from the same origin, the sun. They are different, both intrinsically and in the use we make of them, but they come from the same source.

Now we go on with the father of Western medicine, Hippocrates. He was born in the fifth century BC on the island of Cos, Greece, and defined the broad basis of what a doctor should be, saying that a doctor first of all must be an observer. Hippocrates taught observation of the patient and, from that, the evaluation of the symptoms. He established the diagnosis of disease. He set up the prognosis or the observation of the evolution of the disease. Moreover, he established something very important, the treatment of illness according to two principles: *contraria contrariis curantur* (opposites are cured by opposites) and *similia similibus curantur* (similars are cured by similars). The law of the opposites is what allopathic or conventional medicine uses as its basis, while nonconventional medicine, such as homeopathy, is based on the law of similars. Each system has its own pattern that cannot be combined with or analyzed with the pattern of the other system. We cannot analyze homeopathy with the pattern of allopathic medicine because their principles are opposite. So we cannot analyze a patient from the point of view of the law of the opposites if what we want to do is to treat him with homeopathy. If we do a homeopathic clinical history, we base it on the law of similars and on everything I am going to explain later on. If we do it with the allopathic point of view we use the law of opposites, which is strictly based on the physical aspect. Hahnemann applies the doctrine of utility: a patient is considered healthy when he is able to use his mind and body to achieve the highest aims of his existence (paragraph 9). The patient's health is rooted there.

Similia similibus curantur

Now I would like to explain how the basic elements, the foundation of homeopathy, appeared. The principle of *similia similibus curantur* forms the basis of homeopathy.

Galen was the founder of the pharmacology that is still in use today. He was a very intellectual person, an erudite, endowed with a great imagination, and established healing procedures based on hypotheses. He was the founder of the polypharmacy based only on the law of the contraries, whose doctrine has prevailed for 1500 years.

Paracelsus was born in the fifteenth century in Switzerland. He was a son and nephew of doctors and alchemists, which is very important because alchemists had a profound knowledge of the energy of matter. He created biological chemistry and introduced one of the most important principles: the law of similars. According to this principle, later confirmed through experience, very low doses of the same substance that creates the disease in a healthy person can also cure it.

The other important concept is *vis naturae medicatrix*, which is the curative power of nature, the capacity of any living being to recover its well-being, to cure itself. It is what we also call homeostasis. We all know that if something enters our eyes they automatically produce tears to get rid of it. If something impacts the body, the body goes even a little further: it creates mucous to envelop it and isolate in order to be able to protect the organism and preserve its integrity. If you cut yourself, the organism knows how to cure itself: it knows that first of all it has to stop the bleeding, and so on. Then scarring depends on what kind of wound it is – whether deep or superficial – and also on the capacity of each individual to completely recover by himself. This is *vis naturae medicatrix*, one of the most important principles of homeopathy. We use this concept to optimize homeopathic substances or remedies.

Coming back to the law of *similia similibus curantur*, since here we are talking in the framework of mental diseases, it is relevant to note how already Hippocrates utilized the root of mandrake to cure mental disorders. He had seen that when given in small doses, it could cure the same people who got intoxicated by taking it and would enter into a state of mania or mental illness. So we can see that Hahnemann developed homeopathy, but he drew on the classics. This is like the popular saying that the stain of a blackberry can be removed with a green blackberry.

Hahnemann was a German doctor who was born in 1755 in Meissen, Germany, and died in Paris in 1843. He was a classic doctor of his time and was deeply frustrated by seeing patients dying, seeing how his colleagues were treating them, the tools they were using, the resources they had for curing illnesses. He was really very erudite, an alchemist with a profound knowledge of the energy level. He was a Freemason and knew seven languages. He left the practice of medicine and started to study and to translate the classics. Finding in classical books and manuscripts statements that were not clear, he started to do research in his laboratory, initially focusing on malaria. The first remedy he developed was quinine, from the bark of the *Cinchona officinalis*, a tree from Peru. He read in a classical manuscript that *Cinchona* had the power to cure malaria because of its bitter taste. But in other books he saw that ipecac (ipecacuanha), another bitter plant that we also use as homeopathic remedy, cannot cure malaria. It did not make much sense to him, so he began to use small doses – that he called drachmas – of *Cinchona* on himself. What happened is that he started to experience the symptoms of malaria. He found that very interesting and tried to do it with a lot of other substances. Drawing from his personal experiences and those of his group of students, he started to write books about everything he was finding out through his empirical study, through pure experience and observation. He wrote several books: *Materia Medica Pura*, *Chronic Diseases*, and *The Organon of the Healing Art* (of which six editions have been published, the last postmortem, in 1923). The *Organon* is one of the most important manuals for homeopaths. In it Hahnemann explains what the doctor has to do to be able to cure patients. He describes it in what we call paragraphs. In my presentation I will use several of these paragraphs so that you can understand what he meant.

In the first paragraph Hahnemann says something that is very evident: "The physician's high and only mission is to restore the sick to health, to cure." It is very evident, but nowadays it is difficult to do it with allopathy. How is this way of curing? "The highest ideal of cure is rapid, gentle and permanent restoration of the health" (paragraph 2). So it must not be something only temporary, functioning just in the present moment. When you have been administrated the medicine, it must be long-lasting and gentle, without side effects, so that it does not cause more suffering for the patient.

The third paragraph is the most important for the homeopathic view because in it is rooted the law of similars. It says that the physician has to perceive with clarity what he must cure in each case and also know, study and perfectly understand what is curative in the substance that we call a remedy. I'll later explain how we get to know the curative power of each substance.

To summarize, then, the sole mission of the doctor is to cure, to reestablish health. The job of the homeopath makes no sense if it is not aimed at reestablishing the health of his patient. The patient is healthy when he is able to choose, at least within the framework of his life, in a useful and good way. This is the best indicator to evaluate the state of health of each patient and evaluate the efficiency of the remedy we administrated or prescribed.

Disease

What is disease? It is a dynamic alteration that manifests through symptoms and signs that we can see in each patient. The observer, free of judgment (we could say in a state like a white paper), will be able to see with clarity what is peculiar, notable, extraordinary in each patient and this is what we are going to cure on a homeopathic level. We are *not* going to cure the diagnosis of the disease: we cure the patient or, better said, the patient cures himself through the medication or the remedy we give him, thanks to *vis naturae medicatrix*. So we cure the patient, we do not cure the disease – the allopathic disease I mean, the diagnosis.

Paragraph six of the *Organon* says: "The unprejudiced observer, [...] takes note of nothing in every individual disease, except the changes in the health of the body and of the mind. [...] All these perceptible signs represent the disease in its whole extent."

Each person has his own way to be healthy, so what we have to evaluate are the changes we see with respect to his healthy state, not the changes we *think* he *should* have. Changes in the body and in the mind. This set of symptoms and signs that you can concretely perceive represents the whole of the disease. That is exactly what we are going to cure on the homeopathic level.

Paragraph 265 of the *Organon* says: "It should be a matter of con- science with the physician to be thoroughly convinced in every case that the patient always takes the right medicine and therefore he must give the patient the correctly chosen medicine prepared, moreover, by himself." Why does Hahnemann add this? Because he used alchemy and alchemy is what gives the curing power to the medicine.

Doctrine of Utility Applied to Homeopathy

Why did I start with the doctrine of Swedenborg? Because we can per- fectly apply his doctrine of utility to homeopathy. Patients are healthy when they can be useful. Homeopaths are acting correctly when they are useful for their patients. The remedy is a substance that we can find in nature. In itself it is not useful, it is useful when we take it and try to concretely treat a specific person. As Hahnemann says in paragraph 22, no disease exists if it does not express itself through symptoms and signs. This is the basis of homeopathy and is also the basis of Swedenborg's philosophy.

The most valuable point of Swedenborg's philosophy is that he says that there are two different ways of interaction between two entities and they do not need to be conciliated, each having its own value and application. This means it is not necessary to evaluate homeopathy on the basis of allopathic concepts. He calls these modes of interaction continuities. These continuities are direct and function according to the laws of nature because they work on the same level. This is the knowledge of the level of diagnosis of diseases as we understand it in allopathy. For example, the appearance of an edema has a direct causal relation with a heart problem. We can understand this at a physiological level; we know it is like this because of the physiological laws. But there exist relations and connections that are not direct and work according to other mechanisms, most of them still unknown. This mechanism of connection is called "correspondence." We can say that a patient, for example, has stomach acidity, or heartburn, and that he also has an acidic character. This reflects the law of correspondence. The allopathic diagnosis will be gastritis that produces heartburn, so the doctor prescribes a drug, an antacid, and the patient can remove this heartburn, but only that, because the drug does not work against the acidic character. As homeopaths, what key do we use to know how to prescribe the most appropriate homeopathic remedy for such a person? We look at this kind of correspondence, this peculiarity, which is *specific* to the patient and, in itself, is not the diagnosis. Gastritis generally provokes heartburn. We, as homeopathic doctors, do not take this general term as the essential or key criterion for prescribing a remedy, as I will explain later on.

The doctrine of utility, at least in its underlying principle, can also be seen in the concept Hahnemann had of diseases: just as goodness does not exist unless it is expressed through utility, in the same way no disease exists unless it is expressed by signs and symptoms. Signs and symptoms are not the disease, they are the *expression* of something underlying. The disease is an inner, dynamic, profound alteration that cannot be perceived except through the physical manifestation – what we call materialization of the disease – of the signs and symptoms. And these, yes, are observable. The patient is healed when all symptoms have disappeared, and by symptom we mean something peculiar.

The Remedy

Now, what is a remedy? It is a substance that can be found in nature. Both the most insignificant and the most toxic and dangerous substances have the power to cure diseases that affect humanity. This is the utility of the remedy. The healing power of remedies cannot really be perceived per se; it can only be perceived through a careful observation of the alteration, of the changes that are brought about in the health of the human body. Only when we observe this power of action through the signs caused by its action on our state of health, the natural substance is transformed into a homeopathic remedy. Only when we ingest a substance and see the symptoms it produces in a healthy person we will know what the healing power of that substance is.

Wenda Brewster is a contemporary homeopathic doctor. In an interview in *The American Homeopath* in 1995 she explained the two forms of knowledge, also described in the sixth edition of the *Organon*. One is called *wissen*, the intellectual study done through reading, through books, and the other is *kenntnis,* a profound knowledge acquired through experience. Experience is something that accumulates as the days go by – intellectually as well. The difference between intellect and experience is that experience is an immersion; it is physical, it is something that our body experiences with all our senses. And we know that what we learned with our body is going to last maybe for all of our life.

The Homeopathic Remedy

What is a homeopathic remedy? It is a substance that has been triturated, diluted, and dynamized. How can we study, how can we have
really deep and extensive knowledge of the substances we use as remedies?

First of all we have to study the characteristics of the substances
in nature: it can be a plant, a mineral, an animal, a fungus, we have
substances in all kingdoms. We are most familiar with the three common
kingdoms: animal, mineral, and vegetable. So we know, for example,
how a plant reproduces, how it is grafted, whether it produces flowers,
what environment it grows in more easily, what kind of animals can eat
it, what kind of plants can invade it, whether it contains toxic substances,
alkaloids, whether it is hallucinogenic, and how it impacts human beings.
This is what we know as toxicology, the knowledge of substances in
their nature. Recently Mikhal Yakir, an Israeli homeopath who is also
a biologist and botanist, has been carrying out a very interesting study
on the evolution of species and starting from there she is also studying
how we can extend our knowledge of vegetal remedies and can use them
in homeopathic medicine as well for what is called proving.

Proving is a method based on strictly established principles and is
carried out double or triple blind. Healthy people take a substance and
take note of what kind of symptoms they get. Then the doctor carrying out the provings collects all the symptoms in a big book, called a
repertory. It is a collection of all information obtained through study
and observation. This has been carried out in many centers, on many
populations, and in different conditions.

Another way to know the remedies is through trituration to the C4
level. It is something that I would recommend to anyone interested. I am
personally very interested and I do it in my consultations. It is done in
a group. We grind a substance that nobody knows except for the person
who is bringing it, add lactose and we experience, not necessarily in a
meditation state but observing each other. We can also talk and I think
what you can perceive is very interesting because we pass through all

the levels that I am going to talk about later on. It is something new in homeopathic medicine; it serves to understand the patient better. The experience of this triturating to the C4 level is, I think, a healing experience because at this level the healing essence of the substance appears.

Clearly, we also have all the clinical experience we get through signs. For example, we know through history that many shepherds suffering from arthritis used to put their hands or feet on, or pick up, *Urtica urens* (stinging nettles). If you look at them you can see that nettles possess some sort of small crystals: they produce a reaction of inflammation and itching in the body, and a feeling of burning. We are going to see that later in the next slide.

Where do we find all of this intellectual and experienced knowledge? Basically in the repertory, a big book that looks like a huge dictionary (we also have an electronic version now). We look there for the symptoms: the symptoms of the patient, not of the disease. We also find provings in other texts like Hahnemann's *Materia Medica Pura* based on zoology, botany, toxicology, and so on. All this is somehow contained in the repertory.

Trituration

What is trituration? I am going to read the description Wenda gave. She says it is "The act or process of grinding raw material with a neutral, diluting substance in order to extract its medicinal powers and render them soluble." "Raw" in this context means as we found it in nature. Another definition is "A dry method of potentizing medicinal substances whereby the substance is finely ground in a mortar with a certain proportion of milk sugar, thereby progressively attenuating it." All homeopathic remedies go through a process of trituration, or at least laboratories should do so because it is in this process that substances acquire their healing power. They are then progressively diluted and dynamized, which is what happens when we shake them.

In paragraph 269 of the *Organon*, Hahnemann says: "The homeopathic system of medicine develops for its special use, to a hitherto unheard-of degree, the inner medicinal powers of the crude substances (we are still talking about a dynamic effect because the disease is dynamic, it changes, and that is why the remedy is dynamic as well) [...] whereby only they all become immeasurably and penetratingly efficacious and remedial, even those that in the crude state give no evidence of the slightest medicinal power on the human body." An example of this is *Lycopodium*. *Lycopodium* is a fern; it does not have any alkaloid, it contains no toxic substance, nothing that in big quantities can really produce symptoms, but it does produce symptoms when we grind, dilute, and dynamize it.

Now that we have understood where homeopathy comes from and what its basic concepts are – what disease is, what the *vis naturae medicatrix* is, and what is the law of similars – we can go on talking about how we take the clinical history of a homeopathic patient.

What do we need to take into account? In the past twenty years many advances were made on how to understand the patient and how to take a clinical history. Hahnemann gave us the basis, but we have to adapt it in order to understand patients in the present. In the past twenty years many important contributions came from Europe, Israel, and India, where homeopathy has become a trend. One of the most interesting concepts for me is the level of manifestation of a disease and also understanding on what level the action of the substances manifests, what the symptoms are, and which symptoms are related to which level.

Levels of Manifestation of the Disease

Now I am going to explain this. Disease is dynamic (I am repeating this concept but it is very important); the observer, free from judgment, takes notes of the changes in a person's health; all the visible symptoms represent the whole of disease.

According to paragraph 153, the signs and symptoms that are most "striking, singular, uncommon and peculiar," that belong only to that patient and not to the diagnosis and that we call "characteristic," are the symptoms deserving to be cured. This is the very thing we need to cure because the physical manifestation, as far as diagnosis is concerned, is the answer of our body. The treatment of symptoms depends on the state of the patient. For example, we can have acute situations, like a patient with fever. Why do I mention this? Because some acute situations have prescriptions that only seem to be homeopathic: "For fever? Belladonna!"

If we look at these slides, we can see that each of these children suffering from fever shows totally different, individual characteristics: one child is basically in a state of shock; another has a terrible headache; another is quietly sleeping; another has eye irritation, like a bit of conjunctivitis; and the last one looks as if he has nothing wrong. Some children are still jumping and playing and are very talkative when they have fever. So we cannot say that all fevers must be treated with belladonna even though belladonna is a homeopathic remedy, and sometimes used also for fever. It must be an individualized treatment. If the fever of this child corresponds to the characteristic of belladonna then it is going to work, otherwise it is not going to work at all and homeopathy will be of no use in that case, which leads people to conclude that homeopathy is useless.

Treatment of Symptoms

In acute situations, such as bruises, insect bites, sunstroke, gastroenteritis from poisoned or contaminated food, or epidemics of influenza, where most people show the same signs and symptoms, each situation would probably need the same treatment. For physical trauma we give arnica in most cases. For insects bites – since, according to the law of similars, a mosquito bite produces a reaction that is similar to, though less intense than, a bee sting – a quite commonly used remedy in the presence of an intense reaction is *Apis mellifica*, which is triturated, diluted, and dynamized bee. This is because according to the law of similars we need impulses a bit stronger than the symptoms and we know that the sting of a bee produces a similar, but more intense reaction than the bite of a mosquito. In this way the organism will react. You can try it; you will see that it works. Another remedy we can also use is the medusa or jellyfish because it also stings and has similar symptoms, but in general the most used is *Apis mellifica*. Sometimes when you get a finger trapped in a door or if a hammer accidently hits your finger – both quite painful situations – a good remedy you can use is *Hypericum perforatum* at 30H. It is instantaneous, after 30-40 seconds pain decreases by ninety percent.

The Clinical History: Elements to Be Considered

When we are dealing with chronic illnesses, or recurrent situations, or degenerative, repetitive processes, autoimmune conditions, we need to consider everything in the patient's clinical history that I have explained before, and above all the characteristic symptoms.

What kind of elements do we need to consider in order to define the symptoms well? We need to consider the concepts of psychology. If the symptom is exaggerated in relation to what is happening outside – for example, if someone is still grieving twenty years after a friend or relative died – this is a symptom, the symptom of grief. In contrast, if someone is still grieving a few days or weeks after somebody died, this is not a symptom, it is just a normal, natural reaction, proportionate to the event. Symptoms are always an adaptation to what is happening to a person.

We also need to take into account the level at which patients experience symptoms and also at what level they are living daily life. Talking about levels, we consider that level number four is the level of delusion, of hallucinations, fantasy, dream, unreality: this is the level where a person who has a psychiatric disorder, a mentally ill patient, is living daily life.

Another element that we take into consideration is when the expression of a patient changes, or when he or she makes an intense, energetic gesture. For us, the patient is expressing something very deep in that moment; therefore we take this as very useful information that we need to explore further.

We also take into account what we refer to as the three laws. They are concepts from psychology: "Sensation and action are equal and opposite." "The opposite for whatever is said is also true." "There is no one or nothing out there other than yourself."

So I will perceive what is related to myself. It means that what we feel, what affects us, the way we take it, gives clues about the "air" we are living in. Therefore we will do to ourselves what we perceive people doing to us, and we will do to others, or to things, what we would like to do to ourselves: victim and aggressor are two sides of the same coin. We live in the land of aggression: one is the active and one is the passive aggressor, but the environment is the same. These are elements we consider when we record the clinical history.

Another important element, as Dr. Phuntsog also said, is what we call the miasmatic aspect, which is the ancestral aspect. I am not going to go into detail here. I am only saying that it is something that exists, that we consider the entire pathological history of the patient's family, the personal background, and, if we know it, the patient's pre- and postnatal history, the prevailing conditions at the time of birth. The patient's previous history is also very important for the clinical history because it gives us clues.

Kingdoms

How do we classify information in order to more easily find the remedy a person needs? This is a relatively new approach in homeopathy. We classify remedies by kingdoms. Each individual kingdom – this slide shows the three main ones – has an experience that is shared, the nucleus of suffering. For example, mineral remedies have to do with identity, performance, and structure: what profession, what identity, what I have, what I do not have, what kind of tools I have in order to perform in daily life.

The vegetable kingdom, which takes into account more the sensitivity and reactivity, has to do with how I live, how my environment affects me and how I adapt myself to it. Just like plants. Sometimes plants do not grow for years but then suddenly they do grow because the right conditions have appeared. I put seeds of lettuce and tomatoes in pots and I observed that some lettuce seeds required months to develop. They need to find the right moment. This is the sensitivity the patient needs in his nucleus: to be able to understand what the situation is and how to adapt to unfavorable conditions.

If a patient needs a remedy from the animal kingdom – a snake, a bee, a spider, or mammals – basically his nucleus of suffering is on the level of survival with respect to others that can eat him, or kill him. Just like animals.

Levels: The Seven Levels of Experience

Now let's talk about the levels: what are they? We have seven levels of experience – I did not put the seventh on the slide because it is the level of nonduality.

On level one we have the diagnosis, the allopathic diagnosis of the disease, the symptoms that are characteristic of the disease and that we can see in most patients.

The second level is the level where the patient describes the symptoms and the specificities of the symptoms. For example, what makes the patient feel better, or feel worse, and how it affects him. It is a physical description of the symptoms but it is personalized. It is a very important level when we take the clinical history.

Level three is the emotional level: we consider it but not so much because it does not really give us reliable or deep information about the remedy the patient needs. However, if the patient needs it, we let him talk.

Level four is the level of dreams, fantasy, and intrinsic fears. This is the level where children live a lot, so when they come to the homeopath it is very easy to find the remedy unless they have been very repressed by education. But if they express themselves by playing, by their social interaction with the doctor, by how they talk, whether they stay close to their mother or stay alone, or whether or not they hide behind the chair, all this gives us a lot of information because children live on the level four, the level of playing, of fantasy, of imagination.

[Level five is the level of sensation.]

[Level six is the level of energy.] I would like to give you an example. In the pattern of energy the *manifestation* according to personal experience could be, as I said before, mineral, vegetal, or animal. Who has not seen a soccer match? When the team scores everybody jumps up, shouting. That is the level of energy. How each of us experiences, that is the level of our vital sensation; that is the level of our profound experience. As homeopaths, we try to understand what the individual's experiential level is.

Case History

In this slide we have an example of a diagnosis, a diagnosis of arthritis. We know the anatomy, we know what kind of elements or components we have in the knees, we know the symptoms, we have different pathologies, and then we also have our radiological images that give us more information. So we have the diagnosis. But what we are more interested in is the symptoms, and mostly the particularities, the modalities. We might have a patient who tells us: "When I have an arthritis attack, if it is hot it is more painful and when there is humidity I feel much better." Probably he is talking from the point of view of a vegetal type of person, of how nature affects him, of how he adapts to changes.

Another one might say: "I have pain. I need phosphorus, I need calcium, I need something because otherwise I cannot walk, I cannot move, I cannot do this or that, I am limited in my condition and capacities." This is maybe a more mineral language. Or somebody says "It feels as if someone is pinching me, as if somebody is actually putting needles into my skin," he is talking more in the animal language.

Then there are emotions or experiences that can trigger a pathology or that accompany a pathological symptom. For example: "When I have a painful attack in my knee I feel anger." And we also use images to describe the feeling of pain we have, such as: it's *as if* somebody is pinching me; it's *as if* a spider or a bee is stinging me. The [standard] response to this kind of pain is to give arnica. Because of this mis-understanding that associates pain with arnica, people say: Well, he has arthritis so we will give him arnica because the pharmacy, or the laboratory, says so. But this is not the case here. We have a diagnosis of arthritis, we have symptoms and modalities that are the deep expe-riences of the patient, and we also have images: *as if* a bee is stinging me, *as if* someone is putting needles into my skin. In the case of more vegetal language, we do have a plant that we know because we have studied it, and it has all the characteristic conditions of the symptoms of the patient: *Urtica urens*. So applying the law of similars, the popular clinical experience, and all the knowledge we have gathered, we will give the patient *Urtica urens*.

Factors that can make it more difficult to cure patients include an occasional reticence to collaborate.

Summary

1) Disease is a dynamic alteration that manifests through signs and symptoms. 2) We need to understand the importance of *vis naturae medicatrix*, the capacity of our organism to recover without need of external help: it knows perfectly well how to recover; it has all the internal tools to recover. 3) There are two different modes of inter-action between two elements: the continuities and correspondences (or empirical observation). 4) The doctor must be a nonjudgmental observer who has the ability to evaluate the changes in the state of health of the patient. 5) There are two ways to approach treatment: the principle of *contraria contrariis curantur* of allopathy and that of *similia similibus curantur* of homeopathy. 6) Disease expresses itself on different levels. Level four is the level of mental pathology if the patient is living his daily life in a situation of delusion. 7) Knowledge of natural substances is a key.

I apologize for using so much time of the program. Thank you very much for your attention.

(3rd session)

Dr. Li Qilin graduated from the School of Traditional Chinese Medicine (TCM) in Shanghai with a degree in medicine in 1987. That same year, she began working as a professor of acupuncture at the University of Traditional Chinese Medicine (TCM) in Yunnan. She subsequently completed two years of post-graduate training in acupuncture and currently works as a doctor in the Acupuncture Department of the Associated Hospital of the School of Traditional Chinese Medicine in Yunnan.

From 1996 to 2000, she was a professor at the European Foundation of Traditional Chinese Medicine (TCM). During that same period, she was also head of the post-graduate acupuncture program, a two-year course of study aimed at doctors and organized by the Tarragona School of Doctors. She also worked for seven years as a professor at the Higher Institute for Traditional Medicine of Barcelona (ISMET). For the last two years, she has been teaching courses on TCM within the framework of the Els Juliols program of the University of Barcelona.

She has 26 years of practical and teaching experience in the field of traditional Chinese medicine and Western medicine. From 2000 to date, she has been working as an acupuncturist at the Barcelona Center for Complementary Medicine.

PRESENTATION

LI QILIN
The Influence of Emotions on the Organs According to Traditional Chinese Medicine.

Thank you very much. I would first like to thank Eva, who offered me this opportunity to be a kind of bridge between the two systems of medicine. I've always felt that both types of medicine are the best way and the way of the future, and this is also what I have been taught. I also want to apologize. I've been living for many years here in Spain but my level of Spanish is not enough to be able express myself and transmit everything I would like to transmit.

The presentation I have prepared is not something that reflects only my own ideas. It is something that is also based on the studies I have been following with the ancient books. This is what I would like to communicate to you. The ideas I'm going to explain more or less come from the time of the founder of medicine, Hippocrates, but it is not known exactly when the concepts behind the basic principles of traditional medicine first originated. Normally they are thought to have evolved in the period between the seventh and second century BC. These principles were not developed by only one author; there are various sources.

If it is still not completely clear after my presentation, some libraries have the ancient book that is considered the bible of Traditional Chinese Medicine. It is called *Su Wen*. Actually, its name is *Huangdi Neijing* and it is divided into two parts: *Su Wen* and *Ling Shu*. It is easy to find in English, in English-speaking countries. In Spain you can also find it in Spanish but only the first two parts of one of the books. I have read it. Several things in the translation are not exactly what is expressed in the book or what this culture intends to transmit. The translation is not one hundred percent perfect, but it is rather good.

In Traditional Chinese Medicine, psychological activities are considered a consequence of a set of functions of *all* of the body's systems, not just the brain as in the perspective of conventional medicine. The brain is the place where the information that is gathered is processed, and once this information has been analyzed it is remitted back to the origin. If this energy, this information, comes from the cardiovascular system, for instance, it is sent back to where it came from, to its origin, completing a global, cerebral systemic process.

Those of us who have studied conventional medicine, psychology, and the like, know all about consciousness, emotions, capacity of concentration, memory, and so on. All these things are functions of the brain. But our medicine considers the brain only a place, an important place that receives information from the various systems, analyzes it, and then transmits it through an energetic network so that the body reacts to this information, whether it is emotional, physical, or even at a higher level, a spiritual level. Here we are concentrating on the level of emotions.

In Chinese medicine we have five systems or control centers about which I would like to talk a little more if we have time. It is a network of energy that we call the energetic meridian system. Through its connections this system distributes energy to different parts of the brain and together with the brain controls the different classes and types of emotions (we know, for example, that the part in charge of emotions is the frontal or temporal part of the brain). This is nothing new; it is an ancient idea. It is what we understand about the anatomy of the central nervous system, of the whole nervous system.

So on the first level we have the brain. Then we have this network of energy. That is the second level. We can compare it to a subway network or a system of roads or highways in cities like Barcelona, London, or New York. Then the third level consists of the systems or the organs of the body. When all these sets together work correctly, then we can produce healthy and stable emotions. The imbalance between the system and the brain, or the energetic or physical malfunctioning of any part of this set, from the organs to the system of coordination, can cause severe emotional or physical problems, or both at the same time. This imbalance, be it a blockage, insufficiency, or even an excess of energy, can involve any part of the energy channels.

At this point we can understand that it is not that only the brain produces feelings – such as, for example, happiness or joy. Each system is in charge of controlling basic emotions, but interconnected with the brain. For example, we understand that in the center of the cardiovascular system, in the heart, the most concentrated place of energy in the body, is an important control center. We call it *shen*.

We have five important centers of control and the *shen* is in charge of all of them. That is why we say that the heart is the most important organ. Perhaps you read an article published in the *Vanguardia* several months ago about some research on there being something like 50,000 neurons in the heart. I really enjoyed reading that because it proves that there is also some scientific evidence. People always say our medicine is not scientific, but when I read this article I thought that now I could tell some of my patients who do not want to hear the energetic part that this is science, that there is scientific evidence, and that we are going in a good direction.

Each of these centers controls [a different aspect]; the *shen* is in charge of conscience, thoughts, and also spirituality. This explains why some people are more spiritual than others. In Chinese medicine when we talk about someone with a big heart, it is a person with more awareness, more balanced thoughts, a person who tends to be more spiritual. The *shen* of the heart also directs and coordinates all functions of the body, both at a physical and emotional level, in conjunction with the brain.

The *hun* is the system in charge of the liver, the spleen, it regulates psychological balance, emotional control, and involuntary mental activities, as well as sleep. The *hun's* role, at the level of the energy channels in the body, is like that of the police in a city. If the *hun* is working correctly, in a balanced way, theoretically, the energy channels are open, are free and therefore work well. And the *hun* also gives a capacity of concentration together with the *shen* of the heart. It supports the *shen* and is energetically closely linked to it. I will explain this later.

Then comes the *po*; it is concentrated and located in the respiratory system. It is in charge of the senses, of the basic instincts – like feeding and self-defense – and also of reaction to stimuli.

The *yi* is in charge of the digestive system, of reflection and motivation and the capacity to create illusions.

Talking about emotions, it is important to understand that nothing is isolated. The energetic network system starts in one place and finishes in another. Energy intervenes and mixes, so emotions depend on the moment, you have a dominating emotion, but it is never isolated.

The fifth, *zhi*, is in charge of the urinary system in general, and also memory. Although we may have memory when we are born, *zhi* is in charge of the development of this memory, of the capacity of judgment, the capacity of analysis and making decisions, the capacity to accumulate and develop wisdom, the capacity to reach goals once they are established by planning and organizing.

One of our ancient medical books talks about how *shen*, *hun*, and *po* are intrinsic or hereditary. We are born with them and they are part of our legacy. They develop very early during the evolution of our life. Energetic information comes from here. There is a certain influence from the parents, especially the mother, who transmits it during pregnancy. At the energetic level, at the level of the blood flow, the baby in the uterus is very much influenced by how the mother is feeling. So the *shen*, *hun*, and *po* are innate and have the energy of our ancestors.

The *yi* and *zhi*, on the other hand, are acquired. They develop later on. They are something we acquire in life and are not already present when we are born.

Emotions manifest in each center of each of these systems. When the heart, for example, is working in balance, the person feels united with his brain and can be happy. This is a heart that loves someone. We say "I love him or her with all my heart." This is a sort of metaphor, a symbol, that has its origin and basis in human experience. I do think that traditional Chinese medicine, which has lasted so long, is a science because it has been practiced by millions of people over the years. So we are talking about the capacity to feel happy, sad, have fun, feel gratification, pleasure, pride, acceptance, adoration, devotion, and kindness.

If we have an imbalance, in case of an excess, for example, we can see bad impulses, whims, search for ecstasy, pathological manias, obsessive love, possession, excessive extravagance. If there is insufficiency a person does not take pleasure in life and depression follows. That is why it is so fundamental to have balance in our heart, because the heart is a very important energetic center with a very precise function, a global function; this center has to coordinate with everything else.

Then we have the liver and the gallbladder. These are not the same as in conventional medicine. It is a whole system, so it is much more than just liver and gallbladder. It is a system that can be compared with the caretaker of the body. Its main function is to allow a harmonious expression of feelings. If one needs to feel rage, it allows one to express rage. If there is fear when facing a particular stimulus, it will express fear. If there is a need to be sad, it will express sadness. So when it is functioning properly we have a fluid and correct expression of feelings.

What happens when there is a blockage, which can easily happen because this system does a lot of work in terms of detoxifying the body and also organizing the harmony of the energy in the body? We have irritation, rage, anger, or the opposite, repression of feelings or feelings that are not expressed. Not just rage but other feelings too.

If there is excessive movement, we have impulsive behavior, hostility, impatience, indignation, violence, and pathological hatred. This is something we see a lot in modern society, so probably it means we all have some type of liver problems, some blockage, because we have grown up in a society where everything is quick and we never have enough time. If we do things quickly, we never have time to do them well, or do things with heart and take pleasure in them.

Let's go now to the lungs, or the respiratory system. If it is in balance, this system allows us to overcome loss, grief. There may be grief but it will not be long lasting. One may feel homesick, or lonely, but all of these feelings are actually limited in time and are appropriate to the circumstances. If our energy is low we have sadness, melancholy, even a tendency toward depression or excessive self-pity, desperation. A person who goes through a long period of grief or mourning – twenty years, for example – is obviously pathological, as Dr. Phuntsog said. This means that the respiratory system is energetically very much affected.

As for the stomach, pancreas, and spleen, the digestive system, if we have balance here we have a capacity for reflection. However, if we have an imbalance, we have too many worries, too much apprehension, a tendency to be hypochondriac, obsessive, feel guilty or ashamed. We can have an abnormal energy level, which can lead to the disorders we commonly see in today's society: obsessive-compulsive disorders, disorders related to the diet, or addictive behavior, because today we have changed the way we eat in our society. These kinds of behavior are even more common, not just because we follow trends and fashions, but because our diet is very much affected.

Moving on to the urinary genital system, it is mainly represented by the kidneys. In Chinese medicine the kidneys are not just the kidneys with the ureter and the bladder but include part of the endocrine system. In ancient China the adrenal gland was not known, however there was a notion of a substance produced by the kidneys that was called *tian kui* in the book of *Su Wen*. So at that time they already knew there was some influencing factor, though of course they did not reach the knowledge of endocrinology; this is something that was further developed in the nineteenth and twentieth centuries. If our energy is balanced in the kidney system we have a reaction when there is a state of alarm, for example. We need to make a decision: fight or flight. At that moment our kidney system produces fear, we tremble, but it is not long-lasting. If we have an imbalance, however, besides anxiety we have nervousness, restlessness associated with fear, distrust in the future, in society or in ourselves, linked to phobias, pathological panic, and so on. We know that the energetic systems are linked to the brain and also establish a relationship of support/control. This also helps us establish the diagnosis and prognosis and take preventive measures. It is like father and son, mother and daughter: when one is sick, so is the other. If we see that, we can make a diagnosis and a prognosis of disease both at the physical and emotional levels. So the relationship between the various systems, between the brain and the energetic systems determines the appropriate preventive measures, treatment, and diagnosis.

The *Su Wen* also describes the concept of disease. Illness occurs when there is a rupture, a break in the balanced flow of two aspects, the yin and the yang. You know the symbol for sure. It looks calm at first glance. But if you really look carefully, you can see that it is a circling movement: when the black part increases, the white is reduced. And it is like a spiral that is constantly turning. This is the law of the universe, but it is also the law of how the human body works.

The Tibetan doctor who spoke before about the four elements already mentioned this. In traditional Chinese medicine, which started in the seventh century B.C., air is considered as the sky, as an element of the universe. Sky, earth, human. In human beings we have five basic elements: fire, earth, metal, water, and wood. Metal is something that is not really understood well in the West; it can be put together with earth because it often comes from minerals. This system was developed in ancient times because that was the knowledge then. But I think that this system is still useful to understand the balance between the macro and microcosm, or even within our own bodies because once we have an imbalance we are going to develop a disease.

In terms of *qi*, the source of vital energy, I would like to add that we actually have three sources. One is the parents: through the egg and sperm we acquire energy with information – today we talk about DNA, about genetic information. Then another very important source of vital energy is diet, what we eat, and air that we inhale. What we can actually improve or do something about is related to the two last sources, not to the parents. An imbalance in happiness makes the *qi* disperse. Rage blocks the *qi* or makes it go up. If we have too much rage we say that the blood comes up, but energetically the *qi* is pushed up. If we are worried we have a slower circulation of *qi*. Sadness consumes the *qi* and then it is very hard to get it back. Fear makes the *qi* go down, toward the lower body. I hope these images help you understand visually. When we talk about balance, the balance is always relative, it is dynamic, it depends on our capacity of self-regulation. We can have a slight increase or reduction, we can have a slightly higher activation or lower activation. However, if in this dynamic situation we have a balance we are healthy. But if the capacity of self-regulation is overwhelmed we will have an excess or deficiency. It could be an excess of yin or yang or deficiency, lower than the normal level. We can have a deficiency of yin that if long lasting can cause exhaustion and degenerative or chronic disease or even death.

Thank you.

(4th session)

Dr. Carlos Enrique Ramos holds a degree in medicine and surgery from the University of Chile (1965) and specializations in psychiatry and Gestalt psychology with Professor Claudio Naranjo.

He started his career in 1975 in Italy, where after receiving full accreditation he began to teach courses and lecture at universities and professional schools alongside his other professional activities. In 1994 he qualified as a psychotherapist in Italy, where he currently lives and continues to develop his professional knowledge.

PRESENTATION

CARLOS ENRIQUE RAMOS
Psychology and Integral Psychotherapies

First of all I would like to thank the Catalonia health authorities for having allowed this conference. Secondly, I would like to thank Eva, Adela, and the whole team that organized this event.

Estela [Aguirre Beale] and I come from the trenches and barricades surrounding the fortress of Western allopathic medicine. What do I mean by saying this? My training as well as that of Estela started from the point of view of psychoanalysis, from Freud, representing the end of the nineteenth and early twentieth century. Freud started by analyzing a person, for example a hysterical, or depressed, or compulsive-obsessive person, and from one particular case created a general structure, without analyzing scientifically and without applying statistical methods. So this was the first part of my training.

The second influence I have comes from my phenomenological training – based on Jaspers. Some time around 1920, Karl Jaspers wrote his *General Psychopathology*, a classification of all possible mental diseases. Jaspers conducted statistical analyses and research in psychiatric hospitals for psychotics, and created a fairly good classifying system that is in use to this day. Today we use a legal manual called DSM listing all possible psychiatric illnesses. It gives each illness a number and a letter. It is useful from the legal point of view, and it is also useful because other psychiatrists can understand what you think a person might be affected by. In other words, it puts labels on human beings. If a person comes with psychotic or anxious symptoms, I find in this manual their letters and numbers, I write them in his clinical history so that the next psychiatrist will already know that he is dealing with a psychotic person and forget that he is a specific and concrete person. These are more or less the origins of the Western psychiatry today.

Between the 50s and the 60s, Gestalt therapy started as a possible way to integrate mind and body. Actually, I think it is the best working Western psychotherapeutic method. But considering only mind and body they forget that in addition to the body the person also has energy, has its own essence. A little while ago, when one of the doctors was talking about homeopathy, an image of our colleague Hippocrates was shown. He was alive more than two thousand years ago. And it looks like he was dispensing medicine, but in fact he approached human beings as a whole.

I am immediately reminded of another colleague who lived more or less four thousand years ago, Tönpa Shenrab, the one who created Tibetan medicine. He was not only a physician, he was a master of knowledge, of wisdom, and created the whole structure of Tibet. He had the capacity to see the person as a whole, the totality of the person. Of course, if a person had a particular symptom, he could read the symptom, but at the same time, he could also read the whole being of the person – as body, energy, mind and essence. With this picture of Hippocrates my barricades crumbled and I became aware that this conference on integrative medicine is hardly about integrative medicine at all. I would like to ask Estela her opinion about what we are doing.

Aguirre Beale: We are presenting our position, which today you have described as being enclosed within walls – the walls of a fortress. And I think that is what is happening. Each one of us is presenting their point of view, but not integrating the one of the neighbor, which is part of what we might be able to accomplish at some point before ending this conference. But until now we have only heard the perspectives that each person has presented, which have been quite interesting, but not integrated with the others. Is that what you wanted to hear? [laughter and applause from the audience].

Ramos: We have not come to an agreement. Where do those points of view I first spoke of come from? From very limited and closed views.

There is one view of the human being as a soul, a spirit within a body, a body that has no value. The consequence is a vision that is being applied in a rigid manner.

There is another possible point of view: the body is fundamental, the mind exists, but we do not know what to do with that mind. The mind cannot be divided, the mind cannot be measured. How can one measure the mind? So people spend their time researching the body, the brain, thinking they can discover what goes on in the mind. I will give you an example. I look at Eva. My eyes, each one sends fourteen images, in total, 28 to the brain at the same time. Why? Because one part sees the border, another the volume, another the color, etc., and this goes to the whole brain. Not only that, but, I had listened to her voice, and now that I see her, in conjunction with the vision of the eyes, I also receive the sound, the environment. I can see all of you. The passage of the senses to the brain takes approximately 10 thousandths of a second. The analysis that takes place in the brain is a little bit slower, but in total, it takes about 20 milliseconds. When I look at Eva again, time has elapsed and when I look at her again, she is not as it was before.

Therefore, what does the brain do? It invents an image through the memories, which could be images, or thoughts, or emotions. And I give Eva an image. As you can see, the brain works in delay. Why? Because in a first moment it has to receive from the five senses plus the mind, all the information. It processes it. That's the second moment. And the third moment is to go back to reality. This is very hard work to deal with, for us doctors. So I ask myself, and I ask Estela as well, what can we do? I have carefully listened to Dr. Li, who explained very well the basic Chinese medical concepts. Yesterday, I listened to

Dr. Phuntsog, who gave a very thorough explanation of how [Tibetan medicine] works with people.

I ask myself three questions, and I want to ask them to the audience too. The conference is called Integrative Medicine. Therefore, I want to ask each of the participants how we can communicate. Because I started by saying that I come from the fortress of allopathic medicine. This is true. But I also have the capability to see other possibilities. And so I want to leave this question to the next presenters, to those who will participate in the roundtable: how can we communicate with each other?

The second question is: how can we collaborate with each other in order to treat the people that come to us, to see the human being not just as a sick person, not as a symptom bearer. Because I can be anxious, or be depressed, but my body might be fine. I can work on the body, I can work with the healthy parts of the person. And slowly, the unhealthy part of the person will disappear.

The third question is: are we – who are in different fortresses – able to create protocols in order to face the disturbances of people, and to be able to apply these protocols, be it in elderly homes, clinics, or hospitals. I would like it if our homeopathic colleagues, and those who come from China and from Tibet, and we allopathic Westerners, could really create an integration, create protocols that could truly eliminate pain, while upholding the whole person.

For example, if I feel anxious, my heart is beating. Chinese medicine works on the plantar points, stimulating them. This would calm my heart and would then calm my anxiety. Another way would be, for example, in Tibetan medicine. It works with the breathing and with yogic exercises. One could do a series of yogic exercises that would calm mind and consequently calm anxiety. Of course, in homeopathic medicine the same can be done through other means.

I will give you a trivial example that I experienced personally. A friend who worked in a medical laboratory had a daughter who was born with an allergy. None of the medical doctors could alleviate the allergy of this newborn. A friend of ours who was a homeopathic practitioner advised the father to go to a skillful homeopath professor. The father did not want to go, as he was walled in – like we are – by Western medicine, but his wife took the child to the homeopathic doctor. In three days the child was cured. What does this mean? It was not a case of some psychological action that cured a person suffering from a psychological problem. For example, if I give you water and I tell you it contains a marvelous medicine, you drink it with faith and you get well. But with a newborn that is not the case. What do I want to say with this? That we can collaborate with our homeopathic colleagues. We can integrate their work. We can see how Hippocrates, or Tönpa Sherab, four thousand years ago, saw the human being: in an integrative manner, and not just as a human being, but also in relation to the environment, to the whole solar system, and to the whole galaxy.

(5th session)

Dr. Estela Aguirre Beale graduated from medical school at the University of Buenos Aires in 1962. She subsequently moved to the United States to study at the Menninger Foundation in Topeka, Kansas, where she undertook her residency training in psychiatry and completed her training in psychoanalysis.

Throughout her career, Dr. Beale has treated patients of all ages with many types of afflictions, utilizing a wide variety of treatment approaches. Her interest in system theory brought her to work not only with families and groups but also as a consultant to organizations. For the last twenty years, impressed by the psychological suffering of patients with serious medical problems, she has been working more directly with this population. She introduced dynamic psychiatry practices at a hospital that although widely acknowledged to be in the vanguard of cancer treatment had not integrated psycho-social treatment for patients and families.

Dr. Beale was Associate Professor of the Department of Psychiatry at the University of Texas and Baylor College of Medicine, in Houston, Texas. The majority of her publications focus on her work with patients at M.D. Anderson Cancer Center and on doctor-patient communication.

PRESENTATION

ESTELA AGUIRRE BEALE
Mental Disorders from a Psychiatric Perspective

First of all I would like to thank Benedetta, who has been inviting me for a long time, Ester and Adela, who tolerated my indecision about being able to come here until the last moment, and the whole committee in general.

I do not think I will fall in the trap of answering the question. Since you said that the question was for everyone I will not give my opinion and effectively close the discussion. What can I say now? I also do not have a formula for integrative medicine. I too live in my own walls, but I can tell you a little about my professional itinerary because in some way it has been a constant search for integration. I won't give you the full story of the hundred years of experience I have, otherwise we will not be able to go for lunch.

When I graduated from medical school, I was interested in doing psychiatry. At that time I had two possibilities in Buenos Aires. One was to work in the traditional system of psychiatry as president of an old-fashioned and inhuman hospital where all the chronic psychiatric patients were kept. The other one was to enter the field of psychoanalysis, which was going through lots of struggles, being split between Freudians and Lacanians. I had to decide what to do. Indeed, I had already been in psychoanalysis with a Lacanian for many years and I was neither feeling wiser nor healthier, nor more balanced. So I was not totally convinced that that was the path to follow. I decided to leave since I knew about the Menninger Foundation in Topeka, Kansas, a small town in the middle of the USA. I knew of it because it had many publications and some friends had trained there. I applied, was accepted, and went there.

The reason I was interested in the Menninger Foundation was because the Menninger brothers along with their father, who originally had a clinic of general medicine, felt the need to start an organization where the patient could be treated in a more integral manner. The idea was not only to treat patients in a more human way within the scope of public and private health care, but also to integrate the person back into society faster than was common at that time.

This was organized in 1945, 1946, a time when few [psychiatric] medications were available. The treatments were very primitive: cold packs, padded rooms so the patient would not hurt himself, etc., and this continued up to the 1960s. Their idea not only focused on giving back to the patient a more integrated social and family life, but also on the treatment itself. I do not know if you are familiar with what they do there, but the Menninger treatment is very simple. The patient was evaluated, given a diagnosis by a number of professionals (even though Karl Menninger himself was opposed to psychiatric diagnosis). Then the patient would be assigned different levels of activities depending on his or her ability. Within a few days, the patient was involved in making jewelry, or growing plants, painting, or going to secondary or elementary school in the case of young patients or university or college if adult. Gradually they were offered all kinds of activities, and the patients participated in the schedule according to their possibilities or interests.

The Menningers were not only interested in giving the patients a more humane experience, which would help them reintegrate in daily life, but also wanted the psychiatrists to understand the different schools of thought of that time. For example, all of us psychiatrists who were working at Menninger Foundation went to Big Sur, California, for a week of Gestalt therapy, or transactional therapy. Additionally, they always had guests from different parts of the country and of the world who presented their points of view. This doesn't mean it was easy to adapt everything that was proposed, but there was always a fairly open mind in order to take in other ideas.

The treatment at Menninger was very interesting because it did not end with hospitalizing the patient. Once the patient was ready to come out of the hospital, if he was not ready to return home safely, he would first go to a place like a day care – which today would be called a half-way house. Additionally, there were families and houses in the surrounding area that would take patients, sometimes for months, provided that the rules made between the organization staff and the family would be followed.

Will and Karl Menninger were also very interested in the penal system. They were able to develop an institution where we all would rotate to evaluate the prisoners *after* they had been to court. Karl Menninger did not believe that the place of the psychiatrist during the judgment was in the court, giving opinion to the judge, because, as we all know, this can lead to lots of manipulations and corruption.

That is not how it was in Kansas at that time. We saw the prisoners *after* they had been sentenced. The purpose of the evaluation was to see whether the patient should go to prison – there was a prison that was managed partly with the Menninger collaboration – or to a psychiatric hospital, which in that period still existed. Since Reagan all psychiatric hospitals have been closed, that is why there are so many homeless in the street.

The Menningers had a major influence in the treatment of mental patients because they would train residents in psychiatry, ministers, religious priests, psychologists, social workers, and nurses. It was like a fan that kept spreading. And I think that the training given at Menningers spread throughout many parts of the United States. In some places it has survived well and in others it has been diluted a bit, but overall it has had an impact.

I say this because talking of integration, this is an example of a place where some things were integrated. Recalling the doctor who presented the project of Catalonia, it makes sense, it is a good approach, because sometimes – I am just giving an opinion as I am not qualified to say what will result or not result – when one starts with a limited area where one can have more control of the factors, like the way it happened in Kansas, it is more possible to develop a certain idea, or a set of ideas. That is why I mentioned my experience with the Menningers, because it was very positive not only for me, in terms of the training I had, but is also positive to see how a group of people could truly change the course of events in psychiatry. And this I saw with my own eyes. When I arrived in Kansas, in the hospital of Hosawatomy, a small town 80 miles from Topeka, lobotomies were still being done, in 1962. Not to talk about how the really ill chronic patients were being treated. It was not that the personnel was cruel, but Toracyn was just beginning to be used. Very aggressive or psychotic patients were put in cold towels to calm them down. After many hours in the cold, they would calm down, and they would be put in padded cells.

This is an experience I wanted to share. But the other thing I wanted to mention briefly is that we are now in another epoch in the US in regards to classical psychiatry in general. It is a time where people are trying to introduce more personalized diagnostics. And this is not what it sounds like. It does not mean that the patient is treated in a more pleasant manner and made more comfortable, but that the patient is studied more completely. Because in psychiatry we base ourselves a lot on the information the patient provides, and that, as we know, is not always precise.

A lot of studies demonstrate that even patients who are not psychiatric patients, but have normal medical problems, do not always report everything that is happening to them or what is most important. This is a very interesting phenomenon. And this of course happens in psychiatry, too. We base ourselves and our diagnosis on the symptoms that the patient tells us about, on the information that the family gives us, and on the information about the patient's family. This new trend of more detailed evaluations also includes genetic studies, following the example of oncology where genetic studies in research like breast cancer can totally change the patient's treatment. So now we find out that sometimes bilateral mastectomies that were done were not necessary since the genetic studies now indicate us what would happen to a patient according to her biological makeup.

This is also one of psychiatry's goals, not to simply give a patient a treatment because he or she is depressed. At best, that will involve an antidepressant. In the US 20 percent of the population older than 12 years is on some form of antidepressant. That's incredible, considering that depression is recurrent, is chronic, and that antidepressants and the various types of psychotherapy tend to have unsatisfactory results. And I think one reason why they fail is that we still do not put all the biological, psychological, and social information together in order to make a more correct diagnosis. So we prescribe medicines with the idea that more or less this is the diagnosis of the patient and that with this medicine we will get results. It is the best we can do at the moment, but it is not sufficient.

Ramos: I would like to briefly say something. We have all the potential possibilities within ourselves. Everything we do in medicine is based on the belief "I am the technician, you are the ill person." There is a dualism here, and it does not allow us to recognize the great potential of the human mind. Professor Namkhai Norbu, who inaugurated this conference, is also my wisdom teacher. He is the one who destroyed my castle, because he made me realize that within me there is this potential, this enormous potential. Not just in myself, but in each and every sentient being. Of course, an ant will have a bit less while we, human beings, have a little bit more – or at least we believe that. If I have this awareness and see the person who is in front of me, then there is a real possibility of communicating, and of understanding that this person has within himself or herself all the possibilities to come out of suffering.

(6th session)

ROUNDTABLE

Dr. Teresa Herrerías, Dr. Thubten Phuntsog, Dr. Estela Aguirre Beale, Dr. Li Qilin, Dr. Carlos Enrique Ramos

Moderator: Dr. Eva Juan Linares

Moderator: We will start with the question suggested by Dr. Ramos, that is: how should we communicate among professionals of different medical visions? How can they communicate among each other?

Herrerías: To be able to communicate with each other and maybe to integrate other points of view, first of all we have to know, each of us, what we are doing and how we are doing it. That is to say, we need to become aware. I think in this first event we are trying to find out what we do in nonconventional medicine, what is our specialty, what we know, and what we do not know.

I, for example, know a bit of Chinese medicine, very little, because I studied for a while but then I specialized in homeopathy. So I do know something. I know nothing, or rather I knew absolutely nothing, about Tibetan medicine. As regards psychiatry and psychology, I have been learning them during my professional career as a doctor. So I think the first step is this: to share information and communicate and to see what are our common criteria. We have said that disorders are energetic in origin and that they express themselves through the body. We talked of the *vis naturae medicatrix*. We have also talked about the opportunity of individualized treatment. So I think that there are many elements that join us, so to speak, that we have a common point of view. This is a good start.

Moderator: Does anybody else want to add something to this question which is actually the main question of this session?

Qilin: We are all here to try to communicate. We are acting like a bridge for the different areas of medicine. However, I think that we should have a more open mind because we cannot do everything by ourselves. We need to look for sponsors, not on an economic level, but the kind of sponsors that can create influence, like great physicians and big laboratories. We are already doing this here. There are more powerful things that can be done, but how? In the modern world we live in, the economic aspect is also very important, to promote communication among the two areas, the two types of medicine.

Moderator: Anybody else? Does anybody want to share anything else? Among the audience as well? Because I'm sure there are many professionals.

Audience: Related to how to have a more integrative medicine, sometimes it is misinterpreted. It is understood as if we should know all the medical traditions possible. But it is impossible to accumulate all the medical trainings and all possible traditions. So maybe the concept of integrative medicine would be to have a really open and integrative conception – not speaking from each other's fortress but from our respective backgrounds – that would imply and apply to all levels of the human being.

It means a holistic conception of the being, which is very limited in conventional medicine to the physical and biological aspects. We need to consider also other aspects. We can see some improvements in the area of bio-psychosocial aspects, but the transpersonal, spiritual aspects are not taken into account enough. We need to introduce *formally* in our medical training these kinds of aspects and this is not just optimistic, it is a reality. For example, we could introduce meditation techniques such as Vipassana in our medical training. This is a way of integrating the spiritual part, the potential we are speaking about. And we can combine that with more formal medical investigations that are required to demonstrate the scientific hypothesis.

So I think this is a very, very important point, where each of us, from his or her basic training, works on an open and collaborative basis with professionals of other branches, of other techniques. For example, if we work in a hospital, we should make possible the introduction of Chinese traditional medicine. I come from a Cuban medical background. I'm a psychiatrist, a homeopath, a Jungian, but I received my training in Cuba. And in Cuba, even at top biological hospitals, we had Chinese traditional medicine and in my training as a psychiatrist, within the hospital, I learned the moxibustion technique, acupuncture, hypnosis. In other words, we did everything, we had a more holistic concept though the spiritual level was lacking. What I mean is that this is the door we should open. Each of us in our own way needs to open himself or herself to the rest and ask for help. If we are lacking in a certain area maybe because our technique, our training, is faulty at the energetic level, then we can resort to Chinese medicine. I think that in our conventional medicine, the energetic aspect is a bit weak – we could collaborate and complement each other on this point. I think this is the way: to see our own limitation and collaborate, and to have access and allow the individual, as a total human being, the freedom to go wherever he or she needs to search for his or her cure.

Moderator: I would like to add something. From my experience, I've been working twenty years in oncology and an issue that I have always been worried about, and think it is common to all of us, is that maybe we should put in the center the way the professional sees the patient. This is something you, Dr. Ramos, have already addressed: to see the patient in all of his or her potential. Then, we are talking about the awareness of the being. And now I think that the topic of consciousness is at present being studied in a more scientific way, but we do not dare talk about it yet, because all the potential is there.

Aguirre Beale: I'm glad you mention that now because in psychoanalysis, for example, the study of counter transference is something that is being carried out systematically, although not very well done yet. Now there is a movement that started ten or twelve years ago to work with doctors and sometimes even with actors who play the role of patients, to help doctors explore more their reactions when they have to give bad news to the patient. To try to help the doctors see if they realize whether they see their patient as a whole or if they give the bad news fast because they are scared and they don't want to deal with the problems, or if they can't do it and they send a member of the patient's family. This is a very important issue and some organizations are starting to explore it.

Moderator: I think this is basic since much more attention is paid to the symptom than to the real evolution of the being in the process of suffering. I think that it is very important to be able to unify. From this point of view, there are no personalities, just the being who is trying to evolve from his or her experience.

Ramos: Is there any possibility of creating a center where we could communicate, work, create protocols, in Barcelona, Catalonia?

Moderator: No, but we'll make it come true. We are trying to develop the Values Plan we talked about yesterday – and I feel very lucky to be there because the rest of the people are much older and have more qualifications than me. We are trying to develop a *plan* and a *place* to make it come true, to make a synthesis and receive all this information. This is the most important, the rest stays in the air.

Qilin: I also think that all of us who are professionals should try, apart from being open, not to be mechanical. We need to try to be like guides to help those who are sick to understand their problem, so that they themselves look for their cure. That is why we are talking about that potential of self-healing. In fact, as a doctor, our work helping the patient is about 10%. I haven't reached the maximum possible of 30%. Of the remaining 70%, 40% is up to the patients. I'm talking about numbers in a mechanical way, but it is an example. What we do is to guide them to know and empower this capacity of self-healing.

Wangmo: How can we integrate within the general healing system? I think three sectors could be involved. One is the public in general, the public at large. Another is we, as healers or doctors. And the last one is education. In terms of education, what we can do is offer people courses in different systems [to complement] what they have been studying.

For example, as the director of the Shang Shung School of Tibetan Medicine, I plan to offer continuing education courses, dedicated healing systems. From time to time I will invite our esteemed colleagues. I think as an education center this is what we can do.

And then, as healers, what we can do is that once a treatment is really not responding in a patient, we can help the patients to open their view to contact or get a second opinion from other healers. And we should advertise the different healing systems to the audience or ordinary people, to let them know that many different approaches are available in this world. Each of them has their own properties, their own benefits or their way to work. So I think when we are talking to people we should remind them that for their health, for their lives there are lots of options they can select or check. So, in my opinion, these three things we can do. Thank you.

Roberti di Sarsina: I think we are looking at these problems from a neocolonialist point of view. We are speaking about what we are doing in our own backyards, how clever we are, and what we have done. Fantastic! But the problem is that 99 percent of the people have no such possibilities, have no such money, have no such information. So, in my opinion, the term integrative medicine is very dangerous, because it has been misused, or abused, or confused with other things. We must decide or must realize that the majority of the world lives on half a US dollar a day. So it is quite impossible to heal them without being aware of their condition. In my mind the main goal of Hahnemann is expressed in the ninth paragraph of *Organon*: the definition of what is health. Health is useful, is valuable, because we need it to realize the higher goal of our existence. So depending on which values we ascribe, or how we consider other people, we will have a vision of how to face the problem of humanity. For example, going with a WHO group to Africa, we organized a place for access to a water supply. But the WHO people built those water tanks on a hill where the local people have their own [religious] images, and they will never go there. Western people did not respect them, so they have clean water that is not used because the tanks are built on a holy hill.

This small example is just to say how we must respect *their* condition, *their* situation, *their* needs, not through our eyes but through *their* eyes. When you are dying because you have nothing to eat, I can't go to you and say we have to do integrative medicine because we are so clever, so wise. No. In my opinion we need to help people to be aware and especially in Westernized cultures, to avoid pollution and heavy adverse effects of pharmaceuticals, to help people struggle against health inequalities. This is the main goal. Because we are very lucky here. But outside of here there are a lot of unemployed people, with no medicine, no money, and so no chances to get to a private psychotherapist. The public health vision is most important because we are looking to help the majority of people and not a few people compared to the total world population. I don't mean that what we are doing is not valuable. On the contrary, we must be aware that the global situation has almost been destroyed by Western culture – by pollution, by war in Africa or the Middle East in order to get gasoline, and so on. So we have a lot of responsibility and the more we are aware, the more we have the responsibility to let people understand what is the situation, in order to gain their human right to health. *This* is integrative medicine. Thank you.

Aguirre Beale: That was well spoken and you have a point, but I don't think it has to do with integrative medicine. It has to do with public health. If there is someone here who works in public health, welcome! The mission of a doctor is not the same as politicians, or sociologists, or social workers. If there are people here who want to work for the WHO, it is always a possibility. I don't know how many vacancies there are, and I don't think it is easy getting in, but we can work on that. You can always try and later do that kind of job. But I don't see that the work of a doctor, therapist, psychologist, oncologist, of whatever medical profession, is the same work that politicians do. That is a political position, that's why we vote, though our politicians just do what *they* want. Anyway, this is just my opinion.

Moderator: Dr. Roberti, would you like to say anything?

Roberti di Sarsina: Thank you for your reply. Yes, I do not mean that I have forgotten the Hippocratic oaths. This occasion, this event, is quite useful in order to share visions. For example, in his letter to the Corinthians, St. Paul more or less wrote that even if I could understand and know every language and every philosophy and were able to move the mountains, if I have no charity I have nothing. And this, in my opinion, is the basis of the medical mission. In a multidimensional, interdisciplinary vision of health care, we might or we must use any tools in order to improve the social awareness, because the competent authorities must understand and must listen to people's needs. Not to what the doctors say. Doctors have also a social and ethical responsibility, through their knowledge and their skills, to help people. Not only to help people heal according to our various professions, such as oncology or psychiatry, but also by being in one heart, one mind – not one brain. As Albert Camus wrote: "Each new generation wants to change the world. Our generation must try to not have our world destroyed." Thank you.

Moderator: I think we'll stay on this question, which for me is the most important one. I don't know if I can make a summary, but I think that what we are talking about here is really about developing our heart. That is to say, we are all in a learning and evolutionary process of our consciousness and here we are all sharing it. And this is really integrative.

I would like to share something else in this debate that is really political, this Values Plan. Here, in Catalonia, one of the risks is the loss of public health, this is one of the reasons why a group of professionals are pushing this Values Plan. And it really is a political issue, but overall is a consciousness issue. For everyone.

Ramos: Each one of us and each group has his or her opinion and his or her way of seeing the world, politics, medicine. In the human cell, any kind of cell (which we can consider much like an egg), the yolk is the DNA in the nucleus, and the white is the cytoplasm, the ribosome, the ribonucleic acid. A long time ago we believed that one gene produced one effect. That was left behind some years ago and all the genetic industries in Silicon Valley that were trying to work on those basis fell apart, because that concept is not true. There is a new understanding of how the genomes, the genes, interrelate and give information to the ribosome. And what happens to the cytoplasm? The same that is happening here. Suppose that on a plaza in Barcelona some extreme rightists, rightists, centrists, leftists and extreme leftists are all arguing about a problem. Can you imagine what happens? This is what is happening in the "egg white" of the cell when information from the DNA arrives. In the end, the structures of the cytoplasm can either reject the action of the DNA or accept it. And they send the effect outward. But this is after a huge discussion, a huge opening. If we have our own consciousness open, as Eva said, we can overcome the rigidity of our opinions. I recognize my rigidity as a psychiatrist and I have tried and am trying at this moment to open this possibility of my consciousness. Because that is the result of my entire life. The same goes for political parties, religious groups: each one of them says: "I hold the truth" and fights the others. What happens if we start to open the heart a bit? What happens if we start little by little to open our consciousness as Eva says? At this moment we can communicate, we can create protocols together, we can reach out to the people who are suffering.

Moderator: We'll finish here, thanks a lot for all the energy and experiences you put forward.

Saturday, January 11, afternoon

(1st session)

PANEL

Moderator: Dr. Tomás Álvaro Naranjo

Moderator: I would like to congratulate the organizers of the event. I think it is significant that we can be here under the auspices of a symposium of integrative medicine and it is certainly an important topic. We know there are a lot of things to do. We saw this morning during the roundtable how many things still have to be done.

For me is important to reflect on what integrative medicine is. It is very good that everyone has their own idea, it is positive and productive, because it is the basis of a new focus, new ideas, and new approaches, which is always enriching. But the truth is that the term has its history, it is not by chance that we have this term. In brief, the history is like this: the system we know in the Western world is referred as conventional medicine. We belong to it from a cultural and pragmatic perspective, and it is what we will actually find in our institutions, in our administrations, and so on. When we talk about conventional medicine, or allopathic or orthodox medicine, that is the mainstream and that is what surrounds us.

Many of the professionals who use conventional medicine now also use other kinds of medicine. A few years ago we were talking about alternative medicine, and what we were referring to was different therapeutic approaches that were used, or could be used, instead of conventional medicine. That is why we called it alternative: it was either this one or the other one; one or the other. As early as a few years ago the word "alternative" was replaced with "complementary" with the intention of transmitting a different message. So we started to talk about alternative and complementary medicine, referring again to a set of therapies that can be applied *together* with conventional medicine. So now we don't have to choose one or the other, we can complement them. But this definition, too, soon became too narrow.

So now, the next evolution, is what we call integrative medicine. What we are now trying to do is combine the traditional approaches, to combine complementary and conventional medicine. As a result, this means we don't have to renounce the progress we have made in science and technology.

But this morning, during the roundtable, when we tried to agree on how can we communicate from the different fields of knowledge, from different experiences, from a professional point of view, I started to ask myself where this open path will lead. When we talk about integrative medicine, about a medicine of synthesis, we are talking about going beyond a medicine where knowledge is becoming too limited, where technology is useless if we just look at it in isolation. As we all know, certain changes in lifestyle as simple as, for example, nutrition, physical exercise, respiratory exercises, meditation, or relaxation can have a big physiological impact for controlling the immune system, or arterial pressure, or a wide range of diseases, including the ones we are dealing with at this conference: mental health, anxiety, depression, psychosis, dementia. All these things have a benefit directly, not only from a technical perspective or in terms of medication, but also from all these other perspectives.

A few minutes ago we were saying that maybe we should dare to break the mold we are in. Maybe we should start to talk about stranger things than what we have been discussing so far. If we really want to talk about integrative medicine I think that today you cannot be an integrative doctor without being psychologist. If we are able to take this step and integrate body and mind we have to unite different fields of knowledge, but not only of knowledge. My point of view – and this would be my response to the question Dr. Ramos asked us this morning about how can we communicate – is that of course in terms of knowledge and experience, each field, each profession, makes its own contribution. But theory and knowledge have their limitations. They are necessary and indispensable; we cannot avoid them, but they are not enough. Another kind of dynamic is necessary, where a person makes a commitment with body and soul, and really puts his heart into what he does. That is the medicine – or psychology, call it whatever you wish – that we need, and this is where we need to focus our attention when we talk about integrative medicine.

Of course we need to pay attention to the body, tissues, and organs as well, but also to the bioenergetic aspects, the informative aspects, the underlying significance, and the aspects related to consciousness and spirituality. That is what health is. All this together is part of the human being seen in an integrated way as a whole.

So in the end we can only talk about strange things. I would like to invite all of you, not only my colleague and myself here in front of you, but all of you, the whole audience, not to be afraid to integrate this focus. It is something that comes naturally to most of us, by the way. And science, the emphasis on science and positivism that ties us down, should not prevent us from integrating the experimental aspects. We must overcome that restriction, because otherwise we will need many more meetings like this one. And we really must be able to *apply* all the things we are saying. This is what we will try to do this afternoon. It cannot be only theory. What we are really interested in is practical application. And it is possible to contribute from different fields of knowledge, whichever we specialize in, as long as we work toward integration. With this in mind it is possible to integrate medicine with psychology, acupuncture, nutrition, and whatever. But there is another kind of integration, which is more profound and must be accomplished by each person individually. Anyone who wants to help another from an integrative perspective must have first engaged in the process of integration himself or herself. And starting from there we need to integrate what surrounds us: our family, our friends, our social networks but also nature and animals, the planets and stars. That is integration for me.

We are really honored and fortunate to be able to listen to Dr. Ishar Dalmau's presentation on how one can receive this kind of education in a structured environment drawing on the knowledge and experience that is available in this city of Barcelona. His presentation is titled "Integrative Medicine: An Experience in Research and Education in Barcelona."

Dr. Ishar Dalmau has an important role in communicating the scientific and technological foundations of this kind of approach of integrative medicine. For example, he explains to his students what the extracellular matrix is and how there is an intercellular connection on the biological level that is unknown to conventional science. When you are massaging a patient, or when you are putting your finger on his skin, or when you give a hug to someone, many, many things occur that trigger and modify the status of the person who is receiving, and of course also the one who is giving. All of that is part of health and all of that is integrative medicine. Dr. Dalmau will be explaining these things today.

Dr. Ishar Dalmau i Santamaria received his doctor of medicine and surgery from the Autonomous University of Barcelona (UAB) and a doctor of acupuncture from the Official School of Doctors of Barcelona. He is currently an associate professor in the Cellular Biology, Physiology and Immunology Department of the UAB School of Medicine.

PRESENTATION

ISHAR DALMAU
Integrative Medicine: An Experience of Research and Education in Barcelona

Thanks Tomás. I would like to thank the organization committee for the opportunity to participate in this workshop and be able to share this experience with professionals from medical systems different from the classical ones we are accustomed to in our training as professional doctors in the conventional system. And I am truly grateful that we can share this information with all of you. Actually there is not much difference between us; the only difference is the way we have lived. If we are up here or sitting in the audience it is the same, because everyone shares this reality.

What is the aim of my presentation? Basically, two things: first of all, I will discuss what we need to know or take into account before we start to investigate or research integrative medicine in the Western world. As we mentioned yesterday, our reality as individuals defines the context. So because we are here in the West, the conventional system is biomedicine. All the other systems are considered nonconventional, alternative, complementary, or traditional. That includes Tibetan and Chinese medicine, which in their own countries are medical systems in their own right. I will refer to all of these medicines as nonconventional because I don't like the term alternative or complementary, and nonconventional simply means medicine that is not included in conventional medical faculties or hospitals and is not covered by conventional health care.

Secondly, I would like to present from our Western point of view, from the perspective of the society that we live in, an idea of how alternative medicine could be integrated in the West. I will talk a little about my experience at the university in Barcelona, where in addition to learning the scientific approach, future doctors will get at least a general idea of alternative, complementary, or traditional medicine.

First of all I would like to talk about what we should take into account when we want to do research. Everything is connected. Yesterday, when I was listening to Dr. Wangmo, I was thinking about presenting these two ways of understanding medicine. I was thinking: "Well, this is what I am going to say tomorrow." Then the next speaker also said some things that I will talk about, and finally Tomás also talked about issues that I will cover. I think that is because there is a reality we are getting to know more and more and luckily it will become less unfamiliar all the time, less esoteric, and probably will represent the new paradigm in the future. We will stop being surprised that it is possible to have people participating in this kind of symposium or listening to us in other places in the world via webcast, or that there are healthcare professionals who would like to know more about other medicines.

Usually, when somebody starts to do research with the objective of acquiring new knowledge and ways to apply it to solve problems, or answer questions, or explain certain observations, a scientific method is employed. The scientific method is based on two fundamental principles: first the experiment must be reproducible, meaning that any person anywhere in the world can obtain the same results following the materials and methods. Second, you have to be willing to reject your own hypothesis if the results contradict what you initially thought.

In biomedicine, or conventional, allopathic, orthodox medicine, the medicine that we consider prevalent in our Western society, the problem is the disease and what happens on a cellular level. And the aim is basically to understand the physiopathology, meaning what happens to the cells. Then we also want to arrive at therapeutic tools, such as, for example, medication, drugs, surgery, or radiotherapy, and then understand how the mechanisms of action work, test their efficacy and security, and obviously evaluate the costs and benefits of those treatments. But all of this is accomplished in a scientific, philosophical context in which the universe in formed by matter, meaning atoms, molecules, cells.

To understand life, what we do is study it by analyzing its parts or dissecting it; the nature of human condition is dual, meaning the body and mind are separate. That is the method that biomedicine has been using for decades to develop the knowledge that is related with the structure and function of the human body. What happens when illness arises? How can we treat it with the tools I have mentioned? This is the method we use to do basic and in-clinic investigation in order to understand nonconventional medicine, for example, the mechanism of action of acupuncture, of homeopathy, of meditation, of yoga, of chi kung, etc., and also to evaluate their efficiency and safety with respect to nonconventional treatments. To a lesser extent, we use this same approach to examine everything related with the financial aspects, the monetary aspects.

This knowledge is what, in fact, brings us the information about all these therapies and medical systems that are nonconventional from the perspective of our society. But we can never forget that we arrive at this view through our consciousness, through our prism. Ultimately, the question is not what disease is or what health is and which are the treatments to follow, but how we understand what life is and what the universe is for us. In the end it is more a question of beliefs. And it is true because we can do investigation taking into account our consciousness from a biomedical perspective, looking through that prism. But many other concepts that in fact are present in nonconventional medicine are not taken into consideration.

For example, nonconventional medicine considers the existence of a vital energy or vital strength that is the basis or the essence of the universe and what gives us life. And for the most part, this approach does not talk about disease but about an imbalance of this vital energy; the aim is to cure by stimulating the organism's self-curing system. Additionally, the treatment approach is usually universal, systemic, and personalized, very different from the conventional system, which is specific for one disease and then generalized. Moreover, nonconventional medicine has an understanding that the relationship between patient and therapist is also part of the process of curing. Finally, it acknowledges that issues such as beliefs, intentions, expectations that the patient has about the disease, about what life is, what death is, also have an influence on the treatment and healing process. This person cannot be separated from the environment, from the ecosystem, family, work, geographical situation, historical moment. All of those factors are important in the end to decide which treatment you are going to give and whether the person can be cured. This was discussed yesterday in the afternoon talks. All of this is part of a philosophical context that considers the whole universe to be connected and that the nature of the human condition is not separate, that mind, body, and spirit are a whole.

People often refer to the information available to us on a scientific level in an attempt to understand this more conventional perspective, these structures and functions, but they forget about vital energy, or the fact that everything is connected. Based on the knowledge we use to understand the human body, the mechanisms of illness, and the treatments that are available, it is impossible to give an explanation of what vital energy is. Vital energy is not [some kind of an enzyme like] ATP, some physical component; that's not the case. We cannot explain why putting a needle in the little toe can cure a headache.

So what is necessary? What do we need? We can use this foreign model but we need to appeal to other scientific disciplines and paradigms that can help us understand, even not completely but at least approximately, what vital energy is, or how the whole body is connected. In the last few years there have been many, many articles written by scientists, including Nobel Prize winners, who using disciplines that depart from the ones we are used to are trying to find an explanation that at least gives an idea of all these differences between the conventional and nonconventional systems.

For example, to understand vital energy it is now being demonstrated that electromagnetic fields – light in fact, weak electromagnetic radiations – exist and function as intercellular communication systems, just as if the cells were communicating by cell phone. Or, for example, that everything is connected, the science of psychoneuroimmunology. For example, if a person is improving and coming out of a disease, it is because he wants to come out of it and that's true because attitude really has an influence. Or, as Dr. Alvaro mentioned, the famous connective tissue, the whole topic of the living matrix, or the memory of water. And a big step, a leap really, are the ideas of quantum physics that not only address the atomic level but also the protein and cellular level, or epigenetics, the theory that the environment has an influence on genes.

I read an article in *Ara*, a Catalan newspaper, about a study conducted at a center in Barcelona, a pioneer investigation about the benefits of meditation. This work showed that meditation influences the expression of certain genes related to the inflammatory process, genes that are been currently studied as a target for drug development. So there is a direct relationship between the things I do and my basic structure, my genes.

On the level of modern physics as well, systemic thought, system theory, self-organization, and the concept of biocentrism are an application of quantum physics as proposed Robert Lanza, a biologist physician who said that reality is created by us, by our conscience. So all of these disciplines represent the involvement of many people and need to be taken into consideration to provide an overall view of what nonconventional medicine is.

Maybe you know these two books: this one, by James Oschman, is about energetic medicine, and this other one is about the scientific base of integrative medicine. Besides these two books there is an infinite number of articles that allow us to get closer to what nonconventional medicine is. Plus we have new methods to study medical systems in their own reality. This is what we call [the theory of] whole systems. These are methods that allow us to study, for example, a specific medical system including its philosophical foundation, the involvement of professionals, the relationship between professionals and patient, where the practice is done, what materials are used and considering that each one of these elements is unique.

So to conclude, we need to consider several factors if we want to do research on integrative medicine in the Western world – and even in the East, where integrative medicine is also being researched from a biomedical perspective. First of all we must investigate nonconventional medicine, understand the mechanisms of its techniques and therapies, evaluate its efficacy, safety, and costs and benefits through the integration of new scientific disciplines and paradigms in order to build a bridge so that we can use the same language to find shared points. In the end, even when we talk about yin and yang, we are talking about things that from the point of view of modern physics are quite the same. So in the end you can see that it is just a question of language: we are human beings with a consciousness that can differentiate us because socially and culturally we come from different places. However, we value the same things; it is just that we see things through a different prism. After having looked at conventional medicine with a wider perspective, the idea is to evaluate how can we integrate the biomedical system with nonconventional medicine, and what is the best way for a treatment to be effective, safe, and sustainable.

We must never forget that research is a tool to improve clinical assistance for patients. In fact, to quote an article published by Jerry Avorn, who is the source of this reflection: "Researchers need to recognize that different kinds of research serve complementary functions in developing balanced and mature evidence." This is especially true in the case of researching integrative medicine. In fact this image of the Dalai Lama in a biochemistry lab with a pipette in his hand was very surprising to me. It was published in the scientific journal *Nature* as consequence of the publication of two books on physics that link modern physics with Buddhism.

The thing is that based on what we are discovering now in terms of vital energy, that everything is connected, we are no longer just talking about how we can apply or not apply a treatment. In the end it could be that we have to redefine who we are, how we function, and maybe we really have to change everything we are explaining on a level of general training. And when should the training start? Training in the Western world usually starts after your first B.A. degree, when you choose a specialization, [in other words in the context of] masters' or postgraduate programs, even though in many places there is no actual specialty in homeopathy or acupuncture. The best training, actually, should occur during your B.A.

Regardless whether future professionals are going to work in alternative medicines, they need to know what they are, know their advantages and limitations. And I don't think training on alternative medicine should be optional, I think it should be compulsory independently of the specialization. But if we do that we have to change our beliefs. That's why, going step by step, we first choose to make it optional. The Universidad Autónoma de Barcelona was actually a pioneer in Spain and in Catalonia in terms of introducing an optional course for medical students (in physiotherapy and nursing it already exists) where future physicians receive information about the general foundations of integrative medicine, and above all about its scientific basis, in an attempt to find a common language to understand aspects that are the subject of conventional medicine from our point of view. In the end, as a wise physician once said: "The best medicine is love and care, and if that doesn't work, well you just increase the dose."

Thank you.

(2nd session)

Moderator: Our second speaker is Dr. Teresa Herrerías, whom you already know. This morning she talked about homeopathy, now she will *apply* all of that. She is going to give us a case, a clinical case she has chosen of an Alzheimer's patient. Dementia is the other important focus of this symposium.

You know that Alzheimer's is the most common dementia in our society and by a certain age, eighty or above, almost half of the population has Alzheimer's. In Spain there are more than a million patients with this disease.

Integrative medicine offers tremendous possibilities to help this kind of patient confront this disease where conventional medicine doesn't have an answer. There is no medication that can cure it and we don't have a magic wand to make it go away. You already know that we have multiple brains: our central nervous system can deteriorate but there is still our vegetative system, and we have a little heart inside of our heart, as Dr. Li told us this morning. We have another brain in our intestines, and we have a brain that surrounds us, an energetic field with which we can interact. All of these brains are alive in a person with Alzheimer's, waiting to be able to interact.

TERESA HERRERÍAS
Homeopathy and Mental Disorders:
Personal Clinical Experience

Good afternoon. The truth is that I was relaxed thinking I only had to talk in the morning, as the program says. That's why my talk was so long, because I tried to condense everything there. But it is not like that, so now I had a bit of a scare. In any case I will be more brief than this morning.

I would like to show you an Alzheimer's case diagnosed at Hospital del Mar in Barcelona. But first of all let me go back to the last slide of this morning's talk so we can remember a bit what we talked about. I will give you a condensed summary to explain the levels of experience we were discussing this morning in the context of the clinical history. We said that disease is a dynamic alteration that has a physical manifestation with signs and symptoms. We said we know we have a potential, what we call *vis naturae medicatrix*: nature knows very well how to recover health, balance, harmony, well-being. It is a totally automatic process and this is one of the main principles of the administration of a homeopathic remedy that has been crushed, diluted, and dynamized to optimize the *vis naturae medicatrix*. And we said that we have two different forms of interaction between elements. As the famous theologian and philosopher Swedenborg said, we have what he called continuities and correspondences. The latter we can observe, even though we cannot really explain their mechanism of action; there is no physiological explanation. We also know that the doctor, as Hippocrates teaches us, has to be an observer, and as Hahnemann said, must be an unprejudiced observer, able to recognize changes in the state of health of each patient individually. We said that two basic forms exist for approaching the treatment of disease: one is *contraria contrariis curantur* (opposite cures opposite), as Hippocrates said, and the other one is *similia similibus curantur* (similar cures similar), which is the basis of homeopathy. We also know that we have different levels of expression of disease. Psychiatric pathologies can be located at level four, the level of delusion, fantasies, unreality, dreams, and more intrinsic fears. A patient lives daily life at that level of fantasy or delusion. And we know the substances in nature that can become medicinal substances with homeopathic therapeutic potential.

Now I will explain the case history. It is about a patient I visited in 2007; she was 81 at that time. She was a widow, the mother of a son and a daughter. The daughter and her whole family had been my patients for many years, so the daughter brought her mother to my office. This woman lived in her own home (now she is in a residence) with one of her brothers, next door to her daughter's house. In her youth she was a tailor for many years and then she was a housewife. Why did she come to me? She had severe edema in both legs without any apparent cause. She also had a humerus fracture from a street fall, and the neurology department of Hospital Del Mar had recently diagnosed her with Alzheimer's. She had the appearance of a very obese woman, careless looking, dressed in old and dirty clothes, and she was disoriented at the time. She had a history of hypertension, mild ischemic heart disease, hyperglycemia (two acute crises), one urgent kidney surgery a few months earlier, apparently caused by an obstructive lithiasis, probably from an excess of uric acid, and arthrosis with generalized pain. Taking into account her 81 years of age, this was compounded by physical exhaustion, and she also complained of a permanent intense frontal headache that radiated to the cervical area.

This morning we were talking about the levels of manifestation of disease, where level one is the diagnosis based on the typical characteristics from an allopathic perspective. Basically this level is more general and has less to do with the specific situation of the patient. After only one month from the start of consultation, the daughter convinced her mother to go for two hours to a support group for Alzheimer's families to help her to get out of the house and make her do some kind of activity. Since she had the kidney surgery, there had been a marked worsening of her psychological state, especially at a cognitive level and in terms of orientation. This woman had always been a sad person. She was the fifth of seven children, there were five boys and two girls, and the oldest sister had been a long-term patient in a psychiatric hospital since her youth. As consequence, she had to play the role of the oldest sister. As was the custom in those days, she took care of her brothers until they got married. She did not have many social relationships and was always at home. At this point she had become apathetic, showed no interest in anything, stayed in bed until 3 pm without any interest in getting up. During the day she napped and went to bed very early. Two days before coming to see me she had developed this swelling in both feet and could not really walk, so it was a good excuse for not walking, which was something she really did not like to do anyway. When she told me she had spent two hours at the Alzheimer's support center, she said, "I'm the smartest of all of them."

Spontaneous interventions are particularly interesting because if they are consistent with the clinical symptoms they can help us find the homeopathic remedy. If it is a special case I won't give just one remedy, but two remedies. Earlier I said that I'm a unicist homoeopath, but I'm not a unicist fanatic. In this particular case I gave her two medicines. In some cases, such as patients with cancer or degenerative diseases at an advanced stage, or a patient like this one who is taking a lot of drugs, it is necessary to give an additional medicine for specific symptoms. In addition to telling me that she was the smartest one in the group, she also told me, "I never go on the street alone, I always go with somebody, because I get dizzy when I am on the street." She had a strong sense of insecurity, she needed the company of someone else and this was repetitive. "I can't sleep well at night," she said. "I dream a lot. I jump over a mountain, I jump into the water, I am drowning and then I get out and end up not drowning. I also dream that I fall down." This shows that this patient's main focus was her fear and her fantasies related to falling down as well as her actual experience of falling.

So we are now talking about the second level, where the peculiarities of the individual case start to appear. These are the things we have to take into consideration because they will give us the nucleus, the essence, what Hahnemann called "what is to be cured" in each patient. The unique and specific characteristics peculiar to each patient represent the nucleus of the illness. She said, "I have a delicate fine skin and the salty sea air damages my skin." It is a curious statement. It can or cannot be considered, but it has some relationship with the substance that I gave her. During the interview she mixed reality with fantasy. She told me real things and things that had nothing to do with reality, like: "I went out to dance," or "I was arguing," or "I went shopping," things that belong to daily activities. She said, "I'm bossy, I like to order people around." Since she had to play the role of the oldest sister, this was not unusual, but normal; after all she had to take care of her five brothers. She told me, "My husband was jealous," which was curious as well, since she said it spontaneously. The daughter told me, "She doesn't like hospitals, she doesn't like to go to the Alzheimer's center, she has hardly any social life, she likes to be at home, she has always had her own world and very little communication with the others." The mother said, "I was a tailor and people did not pay me, we always had economic difficulties and we suffered from misery." But the daughter told me it wasn't true, that there had been some difficulties in the postwar period, but it had not been that severe. So this was fantasy. This takes us to the fourth level, of delusion or fantasy. And this is something peculiar and is part of the core of the remedy to treat her. I asked about her fears and she confirmed that she was afraid of falling. She said, "I'm a burden to my family but I cannot be alone, so they must take care of me, I always need to be with company."

She also suffered from irritable bowel syndrome. She was under strong medication, had been taking two antihypertensives, a betablocker, a calcium antagonist, simvastatin, aspirin, and an antidepressant for many years, among other drugs. She was taking so many drugs for many years already, so the irritable bowel syndrome together with the strong medication and Alzheimer's disease were causing the loss of sphincter control. At that time I gave her *Magnesia sulphurica*, I thought that this was the remedy she needed. Sulphur because she did not take care of her appearance and magnesia, which is part of the third series of the periodic table, because recent studies of homeopathy have shown that magnesium has to do with the patient's identity. I visited her at three and eight months of treatment. I saw an improvement in concentration, sphincter control. She was more animated and calm and the headache disappeared, so I maintained the same treatment. Then I made controls by the telephone and the daughter said that they were trying to put her in a residence because she had to work but her mother continued to insist that she needed company. She did not want any external person to take care of her, which is very much an indication for the remedy I gave her.

I saw her again in November. She told me that she wanted to be accompanied at all times. The daughter described a visit they made to the hospital, the discussion they had with the woman who took care of her, the visits to the Alzheimer's center, and she listened to all of that with a facial expression that struck me – it was like that of a baby, or a two-year-old listening to the explanations of her mother and just wanting to be sitting on her mother's lap. The patient had many black holes in her memory, she was very argumentative, she didn't want to walk, not even inside the house, she still napped all day, and she put on more weight. She told me all her fantasies. She said she was very rich, that she had been buying and selling for months, that she bought the house they were living in and was busy all day buying and selling and cleaning because everything was in disorder. So this goes back to what she was telling me at the very beginning, the economic aspect, and once again it came out spontaneously. Even though she had so many deficiencies she talked about being tailor, about economic difficulties (that were not real).

For people who weren't here this morning, this has to do with level two, which is related to the ways of describing symptoms, the things that are peculiar to the patient, and level four, which is the level of fantasy or imagination. We have to look for characteristics of the fifth level since that is the level related to the source of the remedy. The daughter explained that the mother didn't want to go to her own house, she only wanted to be with her because she, the mother, was pregnant, and she said, "It is a girl and her name will be..." Then she said the name of her nephew and added, "I need to say a prayer because otherwise I will not be able to explain what I need." I gave her *Calcarea carbonica*. Ever since then, basically there have been telephone checkups, or visits from the relatives, the daughter, or the grandchildren. She is a long-term patient in a residence, where she sleeps twenty-four hours a day because of the drugs. The doctor in charge did not want to stop the medication, saying she was aggressive, but in reality she had never shown aggressiveness, only anxiety about being among unknown people in an unknown place, where she was obligated to take medication that she didn't want to take. She only wanted to take the medication she had already been taking for many years and the homeopathic remedy. After several discussions with the doctor in charge, even writing to him two letters asking him to observe if there were some improvements after homeopathic treatment, the daughter decided to exercise her authority to have the medication discontinued. I continued to check on her by telephone. I am still treating her with *Calcarea carbonica*. The nucleus of *Calcarea carbonica* matches a patient who needs to always be in the same environment because it makes her or him feel safe; the patient wants to stay home like a two-year-old baby, needs to have company, attempts to make some steps, but only if the mother is watching. So its fundamental nucleus is about survival at the most basic level, including things like food, warmth, and economic needs. Patients who need *Calcarea carbonica* in general are very concerned about the future and the financial situation at home. Economy gives them security. These patients anticipate, that is why they think about these problems. So in this case, the nucleus is like a little girl who had economic concerns, which is characteristic of patients who need *Calcarea carbonica*. This remedy is half mineral half animal, because it is made from the middle of the shell of the oyster, and curiously the patient referred to the sea, which may be only anecdotal. I also gave her *Helleborus niger*, a medicine that is prescribed when there is a mental pathology of a manic type with certain aggressiveness. The patient showed significant improvement, the extra drugs were eliminated, the insomnia disappeared, she was able to have normal conversations although she was between reality and fantasy. It has been several months since I have spoken with the family, but the progression of the disease has been very slow, much slower than expected. And she still follows the prescribed treatment. Thank you.

(3rd session)

Moderator: As Dr. Dalmau stated in his allegory, a microscope aids us in seeing and learning much about things that are minutely small, but more useful to us would be a telescope, because it would broaden our view so that we might integrate our knowledge and techniques into our understanding. Very often, people who do not have a complete knowledge of the paradigm of integrative medicine criticize it for not having enough scientific evidence. It is important to address that criticism, because in reality what integrative medicine is offering is more science, not less. For example, we must know the effects of diet on our physical and emotional states. We must know also that with physical exercise we are able to change the genetics of our organism and free up neurotrophic agents that have a fundamental importance in treating certain mental conditions such as depression and anxiety.

We must be cognizant of what these last forty or fifty years of medicine have taught us. The focus has been on genetics, and it is important to take advantage of the enormous efforts that have been made, and be cognizant of what we now know. But the genetic paradigm is not generally supported, because genes are not self-emergent. We know that the relaxation exercises that Dr. Dalmau taught us as well as physical exercises and other types of practices can modify our genetic make-up. In this regard, we need to broaden our knowledge beyond the genetic paradigm and move toward the epigenetic. We know that quantum physics proposes a series of realities that affect our existence. We must start to include medicine and psychology in this type of research. They are behind in applying the kinds of research that other sciences such as physics and chemistry have been applying for decades. We need more science, not less. Integrative medicine must aim for that. We must research, for example, what effect spirituality has on the evolution of the conventional treatment of AIDS or breast cancer.

The two talks we are going to have this afternoon should prove very enriching and provide an opportunity to get closer to this goal of validating both Western and Eastern medicines. The two speakers,

Dr. Phuntsog Wangmo, whom we heard yesterday as well, and Dr. Sergio Abanades, whom I am going to present, propose a commingling of communication and understanding between two different cultures, two different ways of life, not solely in terms of medicine.

In the Western world, if we speak of "wood" in Tibetan terms, many people would be astonished. But in Spain, too, when we speak of aggressiveness and violence we say it can "put stones in your liver." This idea that when we are angry we put it in certain parts of the body is not so strange. Intense anger can produce, and in fact does produce, a general alteration of the entire organism. So it is not so difficult to understand that liver, wood, and anger are related.

Also, if we speak of "fire," from a certain perspective it does not mean so much in Western terms. But if we speak of heart, of love, warmth, affection, and joy, it is not so strange that this emotional warmth, this closeness with our loved ones that produces a feeling of warmth, is related to the "fire" they speak of in non-Western medical systems. And an excess of fire can be a cause of mania. Where would we put this excess of joy if not into the mania?

And if we talk about "earth" and spleen, or "metal" and sadness, or if we talk about fear, where are we going to put fear? In our kidneys, in our bones. Science has proved that when we have fear, all of our cells are affected by it. When we are sad all the cells of our kidneys, our bones, and our lungs are also influenced by this sadness. When we are joyful, structurally our DNA proteins in every cell of our body begin to function in a different way that is not possible when we are constricted by fear, or sadness, tension, and stress.

So these two messages are absolutely coherent and scientifically based, they just use a different type of terminology. Dr. Phuntsog Wangmo's talk is entitled "The Treatment of Mental Disorders from the Point of View of Tibetan Medicine."

PRESENTATION

PHUNTSOG WANGMO
The Treatment of Mental Disorders
According to Tibetan Medicine

Thank you. Good afternoon. I am truly honored, once again, to be here to share with you some of the basic tenets of Tibetan medicine. I have very much enjoyed listening to the other speakers and their excellent presentations.

Today I will speak about how Tibetan medicine understands and treats mental diseases.

Before we get started, I would like to give a short explanation of why the Shang Shung Institute and I have chosen this topic for this symposium. Mental diseases were quite rare in the past, but today are becoming increasingly commonplace. It is understandable that people who are very stressed or have other conditions of imbalance can have mental illnesses. However, ordinary people should not have to suffer mental diseases. In these times, we see not only adults, but also children suffering from mental disease. So we chose this topic in an effort to find some clarity. How can we explain this rise in the incidence of mental illness? How can we treat it?

Yesterday Chögyal Namkhai Norbu and this morning Dr. Thubten Phuntsog mentioned that Tibetan medical theory is based on the five elements. In Tibetan medicine the five elements are fundamental. In Buddhism, in Tibetan medicine, and in Tibetan culture we believe that all phenomena are composed of the five elements. Both outer phenomena and the inner nature of the individual are composed of the five elements. When the five elements of the body are in balance everything works harmoniously. When they are out of balance, things do not work so well. This applies not only to the bodies of sentient beings, but we can see it in the outer world around us as well. We have earthquakes, fires, and floods. Climates that once were warm today are cold, and vice versa. All of this is due to the elements being out of balance according to the view of Tibetan culture and study.

The five elements composing the body can be imbalanced in numerous ways, depending on the cause. As we said yesterday, diet, behavior, seasonal changes, provocations, and so forth can all influence the state of balance of the elements. In general, Tibetan medicine divides the causes of diseases into two parts: long-term causes of diseases and short-term causes of diseases. We can also refer to these as primary causes of disease and secondary causes of disease.

Primary (or Long-Term) Causes of Disease

In Tibetan medicine the primary causes of disease are referred to as the three poisons: attachment, hatred, and ignorance.

As the word connotes, attachment implies an attachment to something, someone, some place, in some way. It means that one's level of satisfaction is not functioning, that one has a kind of barrier in the form of excess attachment to something in some way. We can see this in the example of falling in love and it not working out. The result is torturous. Love, ideally, is the source of or result of happiness, but at times it also brings physical and mental suffering. This results from attachment.

Hatred is easy to understand. If people are angry and yell and fight, the result is unhappiness.

Ignorance is also easy to understand.

In Tibetan medicine and Buddhism, these three are the primary, or long-term, causes of diseases. Ideally, we would control or prevent these diseases from occurring in the first place, but often we cannot reach this goal due to our own ignorance. When we are dominated by attachment, hatred, or ignorance, this can create disease. For example, attachment can lead to different types of diseases connected with the wind element, or *lung* in Tibetan. In English we say "wind," but we need to understand this term. When we speak of *lung*, we need to examine the general physical level as well as the subtle level. If we look at the nature of *lung*, it is described as rough, light, and subtle. Its function pertains to both physical breathing and circulation. At an energetic or mental level, it is *lung* that creates all the thoughts and activities of thinking. So, when we translate the term *lung* to wind, this is what it means. If one has attachment, all types of diseases connected to *lung* increase. In Tibetan pathology we speak of sixty-three different types of *lung* disorders.

If one is experiencing anger or hatred all types of diseases can arise that are connected to the heat nature. In the physical sense, the nature of heat is related to the fire element. This refers not only to what we normally know as the physical fire but also to the energy level of fire. The nature of the fire element is warm, hot, light, and sharp. The function of this heat nature is the physical process of digestion, and the process of ripening or regenerating. At the energy level it governs determination, a sense of self-confidence or dignity. All of this is part of the qualities of the humor related to the fire element, which in Tibetan is called *tripa.*

Ignorance falls under the influence of the earth and water elements. Both of these elements have the nature of being heavy, cold, sticky, and stable. Physically they give stability. The stability of muscles and bone is the function of the earth and water element. Mentally, they provide a calm and peaceful state.

Though they are called the three poisons, if we are able to manage them they do not function as poisons, they work for us, in the form of three energies. We distinguish between where they are formed, where they abide, and how they influence the functions of our body. Why do we call them poisons? In actuality, they are like a warning sign saying: "Hey, you have poison. Be careful." For, example, if we have poison in our pocket, what do we need to do? We need to make sure to handle it with care. If anyone comes into contact with it they could die. In the same way, we need to be aware at all times of the poisons present in our body. In the Buddhist teachings the great masters always say: "Be aware. Be present." What do we need to be aware of, present of? We need to maintain the presence that these poisons are always with us, and not forget. When we forget they begin to dominate us. They become our bosses and we become like their slaves or servants. In this way the three poisons are the primary cause of disease.

Secondary (or Short-Term) Causes of Diseases

To understand the secondary causes of various diseases, in addition to the basis of disease, the three poisons, we need to consider the influence of the five elements. As we have said, we have the three humors, called *lung, tripa*, and *peken* in Tibetan terminology. Attachment results in wind illnesses. Hatred results in an imbalance of the fire element. Ignorance results in heaviness or dullness. These three poisons are the long-term causes of diseases. The three humors are referred to as the three *nyepas* in Tibetan. In the Aryuvedic system they are called the three *doshas.* The three *nyepas* are the secondary causes of diseases. Infinite diseases exist, due either to long-term or short-term causes. We do not truly know how many diseases exist in samsara. Though we try to name them one by one, there is no end to the number of diseases. In Tibetan medicine we identify roughly four hundred and four diseases. One hundred and one are connected to minor or very minor illnesses like colds or flu. One hundred and one are major diseases that are life-threatening. One hundred and one are linked to karmic causes. Finally, one hundred and one are connected to provocations.

Why are diseases divided into these categories? Because even though their recognition is important when we work with clinical diagnostics, the main goal is the treatment. When a patient comes to the doctor, he does not come simply to have a diagnosis, he is seeking a treatment. So, the treatment is fundamental. The division of disease into four categories leads to different methods of treatment. I will explain more about this later.

As I said before, sixty-three diseases are related to disorders of the *lung,* but clinically the number of diseases is not finite. Each has its own cause, condition, symptoms, and treatment. This is quite complex. The sole cause of all disease is ignorance. When you are ignorant you suffer from dualistic vision: me and you, right and left, white and black, yes and no. This is how our mind works. So, through this attitude of "Me and you," and specifically "I am more important that you," we think "my health is more important for me," "my family is more important," and so on. Everything is "I am." I am the center. This way of thinking is called ignorance. This does not mean we should not think we are important. Of course, we have this body and as long as we have it we should take good care of it. What I am saying is that by following dualistic vision, we continue to wander aimlessly in samsara. This is called *marigpa,* and it is the sole cause of disease. We apply *marigpa* in many ways. If you are seeking enlightenment, *marigpa* is the cause of not achieving that. If you are seeking good health, *marigpa* will destroy that. *Marigpa* means not seeing. The opposite is *rigpa*, seeing. What do we want to see? We want to see very simply that our body is composed of the five elements, and that we are living with the three poisons. We must always have this understanding present and watch that. We can also look at it from a higher point of view. Buddha said that all sentient beings have Buddha nature. We want to discover our Buddha nature, but *marigpa* prevents this.

When we talk of mental diseases, *marigpa* is the sole cause. How do we manage to counteract this problem? For example, if we have very strong attachment to someone it can prevent us from being able to sleep; we can lose our appetite; it can cause an inability to concentrate on our studies, or work, or anything. These are the symptoms. We can take some supplements, but the main thing is we need to find what is useful for us inside ourselves. Many people have had the experience of being with someone who is dying. Death is the final destination for all of us. This is not something we can hide or ignore. Sooner or later death will come. When the time draws near, some people are very peaceful, while others have a very difficult journey. People who during their lifetimes had difficulties and were not able to control the three poisons due to being very angry or attached have a more difficult journey toward death. For those who have had a more peaceful or reasonable life, the ending of life is more peaceful. People who had a lot of anger or attachment now feel very regretful, but at this point it is too late. They think, "Oh, I should not have done this or that." How can we prevent physical and, more importantly, mental disease as well as regret toward the end of our life? Whatever actions we perform are done by the body physically, by the mind mentally, and by the energy verbally. We cannot do anything other than these three actions. When we are aware of the three poisons, we can try to control them in any actions we perform.

There are three kinds of negative actions related to the physical body: killing, stealing, and engaging in sexual misconduct. Four kinds of negative actions are connected to the voice: lying, slandering, insulting, and talking nonsense. Three kinds of negative actions are connected to the mind: coveting, wishing harm on others, and upholding the erroneous view that actions cause no effect. So in order to prevent disease as well as to treat disease, instead of killing we try to save the lives of beings; instead of stealing, we try to practice generosity; instead of practicing sexual misconduct we can take some vows or commitments. Doing these positive actions helps us accumulate merits, and as a result we can live a peaceful life.

Verbally, rather than lie we can tell the truth. Rather than gossip we can chant some mantras – yesterday Rinpoche spoke of the power of reciting mantras. Rather than slander, we can say good things or send positive messages. For example, instead of going to someone's husband and saying something like: "Your wife doesn't love you," speak of that couple's love for each other in order to make them get along.

Mentally, for example, rather than planning to harm someone, we can try to create loving kindnes and cultivate compassion. If we practice loving kindness, generosity, and good actions, we can have a peaceful life. A peaceful life is the source of happiness. A peaceful life is the source of health. In this way we can manage to prevent disease. If we try to eat the best things, buying the most expensive organic foods, do our best to exercise, and buy good quality clothes made from cotton rather than synthetic materials, none of these things will work if your mind is polluted, because the mind is much more powerful than the body. Mind is like a king, and a king is more powerful than a servant. So even if we eat healthy organic food, if our mind is polluted or stressed it does not work.

How can we obtain happiness? On a superficial level, if we go to a party we can experience a little happiness, the same if we drink some wine. But it is not long lasting. How do we obtain permanent happiness? Permanent happiness needs to come from inside you. When we have a mental disease such as depression, everything seems dark, like living inside a cave. How can we get light? If you see your inner nature, that is the light. So we must understand that the cause of disease is an aspect of the three poisons and try to control them. How? Buddha's teachings are said to encompass a total of 84,000 volumes. The purpose of these volumes is to point out the three poisons as well as methods for controlling them. This is how we examine the causes and treatments of diseases.

Short-Term or Direct Causes of Mental Diseases

Mental diseases stem from various causes: weakness of the physical heart; strong, unrelenting sadness, or the experience of a sudden event resulting in intense sadness; a very poor diet; and, finally, provocations. These are short-term or direct causes of mental diseases. According to Tibetan medicine, these causes can lead to seven types of depression. We do not have time to examine them in detail now. If you are interested, there will be three days of workshops on this topic.

To conclude, we must be aware of the three poisons and how they are the foundation of our three existences. If we are able to control them they can work positively for us and for the way we function. This gives us a kind of determination or direction and makes our life interesting. When the three poisons control us we get ill. This is why we must be aware and remember the importance of them in our lives.

Thank you very much for listening.

(4th session)

Dr. Sergio Abanades León holds a degree in medicine and surgery from the Complutense University of Madrid. He specialized in clinical pharmacology at the Institut Municipal d'Investigació Mèdica IMIM-Hospital del Mar, receiving his doctor in pharmacology from the Autonomous University of Barcelona (First Class cum laude and European Doctor Mention Diploma) and a master's in toxicology from the University of Seville and in homoeopathy from the University of Barcelona.

The first years of his professional career were focused on hospital medicine, teaching, and scientific research. For a period of two years, he was clinical director of the Centre for the Development of Medicines and Neuroimaging of GlaxoSmithKline in London (the Clinical Imaging Centre). He is also an honorary professor of pharmacology and toxicology at the Experimental Toxicology Department at Imperial College in London.

He is currently medical director of the Omega Zeta Clinic in Barcelona, which specializes in integrative medicine, where he combines therapies from conventional medicine with alternative or complementary medicines validated through scientific procedures and methods.

PRESENTATION

SERGIO ABANADES
Personal Experience of Integrative Medicine in Neuropsychiatric Disorders

First of all I want to thank the organizers of this event. I think it is a day to celebrate, a celebration of the common sense to treat human beings with all the tools at our disposal: with our right hand and our left hand, with our left brain and our right brain, without sacrificing any of our abilities as human beings. This event is a celebration of the fact that we can unite and integrate, that we have this coming together of West and East, traditional and nontraditional. I think it is a day to feel satisfied and happy. I would also like to thank Dr. Linares in particular – anyone who can manage to stage an event from a thousand kilometers away deserves all my respect. Thank you, Eva

I'll start talking about our model of integrative medicine. We are a clinic called Omega Zeta that started in 2011 in Barcelona. It is a center where a few specialists have gathered to work in integrative medicine. First, let me define the parameters of what integrative medicine means for us. We've talked a lot in these two days about what integrative medicine means, and how we see this integrative medicine, but I'll try to explain how we define it at Omega Zeta.

Secondly I will explain our approach, focusing on the treatment of patients and how we combine the different systems of medicine.

Finally I will explain the specific treatment for mental illness, and if there is time I will present some clinical cases in this regard.

What Is Integrative Medicine?

Firstly, for us integrative medicine means the integration of conventional and nonconventional medicine, alternative medicine, complementary medicine, etc., all those forms of medicine that have been validated scientifically, even though of course much could be said about what "scientifically validated" actually means. As we have seen in Dr. Dalmau's presentation, to scientifically validate certain types of alternative or complementary medicine has its particularities. We could talk about that for a long time, but this concept is very important.

Secondly, integrative medicine should promote the use of the most appropriate methods adjusted to each patient, meaning the best of both worlds, the conventional and the nonconventional. In this country what we consider conventional can be one thing and in China, Tibet, it can refer to something different. Whichever is the "other" system would be considered nonconventional. But we are always trying to integrate these worlds.

Thirdly, our goal, and the goal of medicine in general, must always be to improve the quality of life of patients. In integrative medicine we use conventional or alternative methods to facilitate the natural response of our body – homeostasis, the natural or innate ability of the body to heal itself.

Moreover, we also recognize that medicine must be based on scientific evidence. There must be data and assumptions must be confirmed. But we also have to be open to old and new paradigms and innovations. Conventional medicine is based on scientific methods. However, many scientists, physicians, and practitioners of conventional medicine aren't open to new paradigms or even old paradigms. The contrary occurs when we accept everything unconventional without checking carefully what we are doing. For example, if we accept that a person with a fifteen-day training in therapy can put his or her hands on us, we start entering into a delicate world.

I like medicine, it is my passion. But I also like rigor and the critical analysis of what we do, unconventional and conventional. So we are open to all paradigms, but we are also open to the verification of hypotheses.

It is also important to establish an agreement between patient and therapist, between patient and physician. This agreement defines the changes that the patient wants to make in his life, and the level of responsibility that the therapist or doctor should have in healing the patient.

We will also consider all factors that influence health, not only the physical aspect, but also the mental and emotional world. We just heard a magnificent exposition of how the "three poisons" influence health – I would say we have more than three, depending on how we consider them. We must consider individual beings as a whole, because sometimes in conventional medicine unfortunately the more basic levels, emotional, mental, and spiritual, are denied. Conventional medicine affirms that these aspects do not alter or affect our body, but for us, as we said before, they are fundamental, because emotional and mental alterations are the cause of the disease.

Of course from the outset we should use the least invasive and least harmful methods. If we can treat using different techniques we will start with the least damaging. If this doesn't respond, we may use other techniques even if they have side effects. As we know medicine is based on "do no harm." Sometimes therapies are used that may harm more than cure, no matter how technologically advanced they are.

Therefore our model of integrative medicine is a model for promoting health and preventing disease. In [ancient] China, for example, if the emperor got sick the doctor was not paid. I like that, it is a model that really says a lot about medicine, because if we can prevent it is much better than curing. To practice preventive healthcare nowadays is a complicated proposition since the level of stress and pollution we have in our societies is difficult to prevent. Anyway is always better prevent than cure.

Very important in our model of integrative medicine is the training of doctors, therapists, psychologists, the whole team that is in contact with the patient. They try to be models of the healing that we want to see in our patients. We must be involved in our model of healing and we must heal ourselves while we see patients. This is very important; try to follow the model that you want to see happening in your patient and in the people you attend. This is quite complicated, but to a greater or lesser extent, it is applied, because we therapists take the same supplements as the patient, we are doing yoga, meditation, we enter the same programs that I will introduce in a while. So this model, as I said before, is based on a healing team: doctors, therapists, psychologists. We know conventional medicine, we know it well. Sometimes I say: "If we want discuss conventional medicine, let's really discuss it." We can talk for hours about conventional medicine, scientific evidence, diagnostic methods. But if we have to discuss it I prefer to do it with conventional doctors. We are not blinded by our knowledge of science and conventional medicine; we don't deny the existence of other healing methods.

In this slide we have the complementary treatments. As I said before, the same treatment can be considered either complementary or conventional, depending on how we look at it. Our understanding of this model is always holistic. We have to break the taboo. In some more conventional forums you can't even use the word. Yes, holistic! We treat the human being as a whole; in other words we don't view the apparatus and parts of the body as separate entities. As Dr. Dalmau said, a toe can heal a headache. Doesn't that indicate an intimate connection among each of our body cells? So there will always be a holistic way of understanding medicine.

A medical team is responsible and entirely in charge of your health; in fact, if you bring the test results from the hospital, we will understand. If you bring diagnoses we will understand. If you want drugs, we will understand. But the patient also has a responsibility. You, the patient, are going to be responsible for your pathology, for your life. This point is more complicated. We are accustomed to being passive and that the government, the law, gives us everything and even tells us what we have to do. But it is we who should take responsibility for our health.

This is where there are still certain types of problems. But we try to encourage patients to be responsible for their treatment; we ask them to make dietary changes, we ask them to make lifestyle changes. If we want a profound change in the poisons that were discussed in the previous presentation, we have to change ourselves in order to ensure a comprehensive and prolonged healing. So in this model of medicine we want a responsible patient whom we can give a fully individualized treatment plan.

Omega Zeta Clinic

In our clinic, two and a half years ago we started with a team of about ten people. We currently have thirty-one professionals. I am the medical director and I humbly lead this team, with great joy, because we have really put together a team of professionals of a high level in a magnificent environment and with a spirit totally dedicated to the patient. We also have an executive director, marketing specialists, people who handle administration, one nurse – who is here – totally dedicated to the clinic, who is also therapist in polarity and reflexology. And we have eleven doctors, including a rheumatologist, a neurogastroenterologist, an acupuncturist, a psychiatrist, a nutritionist, a homeopath, an immunologist, two gynecologists, a specialist doctor in aesthetic medicine, a pain doctor, physical therapists, osteopaths, an expert in posture, two specialists in shiatsu and Keng Rak, and three psychologists; we also have teachers of tai chi, yoga, and Pilates. This is the team we have created.

Now I will present some aspects of our approach to treatment, which as we will see later would also apply to mental illness. The first step is the evaluation of the patient. We need to take enough time to be able to analyze tests, look at the patient's family and surroundings, determine when the illness first started, and identify the patient's mental and emotional symptoms. Of course we take a detailed medical history and on that basis we always give a personalized treatment that normally requires some changes in lifestyle, a reduction in medication depending on the pathology, and emotional coaching or emotional control. That is also fundamental because as we have seen in the previous presentation there are poisons that make us ill. It's a multidisciplinary approach to healing a patient.

Different hands and different people will touch the patient. Curing, healing on an individual basis is very gratifying, such as in homeopathy as we just saw, but when different doctors are combined, the patient feels helped by different professionals with different feelings, with different approaches, and the results are even better. It's a holistic approach with holistic therapies and, in our case, of course using advanced medical technologies that we have available, always with regular evaluations of the patient to be able to make changes in the treatment. As William Osler said, it's much more important to understand what class of a patient we have in front of us than to know what class of disease the patient has. If we understand the type of patient we have it's easier to treat him or her in a holistic and more comprehensive way.

Now these slides show you what we analyze at our center of integrative medicine when a patient arrives, meaning the social part of the disease. In many cases, it's really important to look at the patient's work and family surroundings, and also the marriage or the partner. Of course we also look at his conventional medical history, what kind of treatment the patient has received so far. We dedicate a lot of time to the conventional history, just as any conventional doctor does, but then we add to the clinical history the patient's life habits, hydration habits, nutrition, sleep, exercise, toxic habits, and so on. We look at the typical family medicine events throughout the patient's life and above all we do a mental-emotional evaluation, paying attention to anxiety, depression, etc. This emotional part can take a big part of the visit. Physical symptoms also tell us what is happening with the patient – many patients come from traditional Chinese medicine. Then we also do a bio-energetic evaluation using the medical technology we have at our disposal. And in almost all patients we have to measure subjectively and objectively whether physical pain and stress are present, because pain and stress can be the cause of any kind of emotional-mental disorders.

When patients come to our center we give them a scientifically validated questionnaire about their quality of life to be able to see what kind of changes we are achieving in their health. We want to know basically whether the quality of life has increased or not, and not whether a single symptom has or not improved.

Now let's look at our therapeutic focuses: I'm not going to discuss all of them, just two very important ones that are linked with our topic – the mental pathologies: our psychoneuroendocrinology and immunology unit and our integral care service for mental patients. There are others, as you can see on the list.

And then the diseases we treat in our clinic: any kind of pain, chronic pain, autoimmune illnesses, arthritis, fibromyalgia, etc. The ones underlined in red are more linked to today's topic: depression, anxiety, stress, and insomnia – something we see daily in the society we leave in – and also the neurodegenerative disease that we will be talking about afterward, and also ADHD, attention deficit hyperactivity disorder in kids.

We can structure the various treatments around this model. We work not only with drugs and conventional medicine, but also with holistic medicine. Of course, we mainly use traditional Chinese medicine and acupuncture as one of its branches, homeopathy, and polarity therapy. These are three therapeutic areas we can use in treating patients for nearly all the symptoms they present.

It is very interesting to consider a psychoneuroendocrinological approach, prescribing natural supplements for those elements that could be lacking, like vitamins and minerals, and also carrying out analyses to see how the gut flora is. We want to detect what is physically lacking to be able to supplement in a suitable way. Another approach is ortho-molecular therapy.

And as far as manual therapies are concerned, very often – as we have seen in the previous talk – before patients can look into their heart and confront their poisons and mental phantoms we need to put our hand on their bodies. Unfortunately, a lot of our patients are not used to being touch, are not used to being embraced or massaged, so first they need to reconnect with their body and in order to reconnect with the body you have to touch it. We have therapies like Keng Rak, Ho'oponopono, shiatsu, osteopathy, reflexology, and so on. We also use technologies like ES-TECK, a scientifically validated computer-assisted medical system for assessing the functional health status of the body. And what is especially important to complete our patient services, in addition to the clinic with all these kinds of technologies and treatments, we now have a facility for Mind-Body Medicine in a small building next door where we can also use the techniques that have been scientifically validated. We are very proud to say that we have increasing scientific evidence of the body's ability to cure itself through yoga and meditation, Pilates, tai chi, and so on.

I would like to show you a brief video so you can see our clinic and what we do. [Shows video.] It is a center, as I said, where we were able to harmoniously integrate in one and the same space conventional and nonconventional medicine that has been scientifically validated. You can see some of our treatment rooms, some of the techniques we utilize: massage, magnetic therapy treatments, bioelectrical stimulation. This is the room we created for Mind-Body therapy; it has very good energy vibrations and we use it for yoga, meditation, tai chi, these kinds of therapies.

Neuropsychiatric Treatments

In the field of neuropsychiatric treatments, I would like to focus on what we can do for this kind of patient. At our center we try to combine different types of therapies, not only one; we practically combine all of them. Almost all our patients have a homeopathic treatment and receive some degree of natural supplementation treatment based on the analyses that tell us what is missing in the patient. Acupuncture, personal nutrition, therapies at an energetic level, cognitive stimulation, mindfulness, and relaxation techniques are fundamental in treating this kind of disease.

The detoxification of heavy metals is a very important topic. In some degenerative illnesses we find the presence of a high degree of toxicity when we analyze the hair and plasma of the patient. We always do a careful review of the pharmacological treatment. Sometimes patients come whose symptoms result only from the treatment they have been receiving: we then have to stop that treatment, see how things develop, and then intervene. Sometimes we interpret homeopathic symptoms as if they come from the patient, instead they come from the treatment the patients are receiving, and this is a big mistake. And of course it is always important to help the family (above all in case of mental and neurodegenerative diseases, which can affect the patient and the patient's family). We have the same model for treating neuro-psychiatric illnesses, from the evaluation of the patient to all the other steps I just outlined, and of course we do regular evaluations with this multidisciplinary team.

I would like to show you a couple of cases so you have concrete examples. One is a case of olivopontocerebellar atrophy. This is a disease that doesn't have a conventional treatment. In this case it was noninherited – some cases are hereditary or genetic. The condition has an idiopathic, or unknown, cause. But in conventional medicine there is no treatment. No treatment, no hope, right? If you go to a clinic and they tell you there is no treatment, that it will get worse and worse, that you will end up in a wheelchair and then die, this will have an impact on your being. It can also be accompanied by dysphasia, dysarthria, above all ataxia, meaning the inability to coordinate movement, urinary and respiratory problems, sleep-associated disorders, and much more. This disease normally progresses until a neurodegenerative state, wheelchair, and death.

The patient in this case was a 62-year-old woman with no previous clinical condition, only a long history of anxiety and depression symptoms that occasionally had been treated with drugs, but only for six-month periods. The clinical presentation included moderate ataxia, or unstable walking, which is the principal symptom of this disease. Of course, sleep was disrupted, she had anxiety, and a poor quality of life, first of all because of the disease, but also due to a fear of dying and a fear of affecting the quality of life of her family (which, of course, made things worse not only for her but for her whole family).

In the second clinical interview with her, I asked about all the treatments she had received. We took an in-depth homeopathic history to see what kind of treatment we could give her. At one point I asked her what was the one thing in her life that was preventing her from moving. She had ataxia, but what was it that was *really* blocking her? So we discovered the main point, the central element of this patient pathology: a traumatic relationship with the mother. The mother, still alive, had suffered from mental illness and had caused the daughter to suffer since childhood from psychological abuse. It was a torturous relationship.

What did we do with this patient? We treated her with the approach I presented earlier. We treated the profound traumatic disorder with individualized homeopathy, in this case with two very interesting remedies that come from the world of minerals that we find in the periodic table that have been recently discovered in homeopathy and that are very efficacious in curing certain autoimmune diseases. And above all we gave her techniques to free her emotions in order to unblock them. She had such rage and hatred inside. We tried to help her be more present in her life. We also analyzed the toxins (we eventually had to detoxify a heavy metal), and we supported the entire neurodegenerative process by giving her ginko biloba, glutamine, thyroxin, and some other highly concentrated supplements together with antioxidants, including high doses of Omega3 and green tea extract. Moreover, we put her on a program of magnetic treatments that we offer. We also did immunology tests and saw that there was also an underlying immunological problem coupled with moderate to severe immunodepressions, and an active Epstein-Barr virus, which we treated with microimmune therapy.

What we have seen is that at neurological level, in thirteen months after her arrival there was no deterioration, which usually goes quite fast. Positive symptoms include an increase in muscle tone; no complications; we resolved the anxiety and sleep disturbance; and above all we saw an authentic, deep change in her traumatic relationship with her mother. The questionnaire about her quality of life indicated significant effects both in her own and her family's quality of life. And above all the treatment has given hope both to the patient and her family. It's a very complicated case; we don't know how it will evolve, but we are very satisfied that for the moment we have clinical stability and an improvement in the patient's situation.

Part of the treatment she has received is a magnetic treatment that is very interesting, a very low frequency treatment. The patient lies on a mat that is connected to this machine and the mechanism improves the detoxification of cells and stimulates the process of regenerating body tissues. We have been utilizing this machine, which reduces pain and inflammatory processes, as a coadjuvant treatment for the patient. We programmed the device and she has been able to take the satellite equipment home (she lives 200 km from Barcelona). After forty days of this magnetic treatment at home she returns to our center, the device is reprogrammed depending on the improvement or changes, and we start the cycle again. We have been doing this coadjuvant treatment for nine months. The treatment comes from Italy, where it is being tested with promising results for neurodegeneration.

I had another case of Alzheimer's but since we do not have any time, we finish here. Thank you.

ROUNDTABLE

Dr. Ishar Dalmau, Dr. Teresa Herrerías,
Dr. Phuntsog Wangmo, Dr. Sergio Abanades

Moderator: Dr. Tomás Álvaro Naranjo

Moderator: We have now an opportunity to continue to explore these interesting perspectives and take advantage of the extraordinary speakers who are here with us to learn as much as we can from their knowledge and experience. I invite all of you to participate, make comments, and open the discussion. Anyone? We have a lot to talk about.

Audience: First I wish to congratulate you all for these magnificent presentations. I would just like to add something to the last presentation of Sergio. As you have said, of course in the clinic and when we talk about hospitals, about patients, it is not typical to use alternative or complementary techniques unless they have been scientifically validated. But research is another thing, and I think that is what we have to concentrate on, because we would not be here talking about this topic today if we had not dared to do things that years ago were unthinkable. I want to say that is very important to research techniques that have not been empirically validated. There are many things we do not yet know. It is a kind of invisible medicine, but it is important to go beyond it and give value to techniques that doctors have not taken into account so far. I think the moment has arrived to put them on the table, focus our attention on them, even though they have not been empirically proven. Maybe what today is magic, tomorrow is science. I would like to know your opinion about this.

Abanades: I completely agree with you. I think we have now arrived at an important moment in that respect and scientific arrogance should not dismiss things as magic. One has to be linked to the other. With a lot of arrogance, acupuncture has been dismissed for many years because we could not believe in it. It is millenary science with a "magical" placebo effect that has passed from generation to generation since the beginning of time. But recent meta analysis has shown that people don't have faith in acupuncture's positive influence on health. As I said before, it is a doubt we have. Or rather it is not so much a doubt as rejection. It is one thing to be scientifically skeptical, another to reject everything you do not believe.

It is very clear that a person is composed of spirit, mind, and physical body. And there are streams of subtle energies that nourish us, that move us and give us life. The study of these subtle energies has to be the medicine of the twenty-first century. We need to study and verify that those subtle energies are what really move us and when they are not functioning we fall ill. Empirical data give us the idea that the subtle energies are responsible for our life, our death, our diseases. This is the study we should explore more profoundly, in my opinion.

Audience: I would like to thank all of you. Continuing along the same lines, in your experience to what extent do you find fairness, honesty, and coherence in the patients who come to your practice and explain their condition? I ask this in relation to what Tomás said, that we start to open up in respect to the vital processes, emotions that a lot of people are experiencing, and always have experienced, but maybe at the moment it is something more cathartic or widespread. And the fact that there is a prejudice about these experiences. This has many names. Some call it emerging spirituality, or consciousness shift, or the connection with *akasha*, the essence of all things. It does not matter the name we choose, the fact is that the mind is free, without limits. And then the mental structures that limited us are starting to break apart. This is where you enter a pure chaos, a pure terror because in addition to the fact that you cannot express what is going on inside of you, outside, too, there is no real understanding of what is happening. At most people could have a bit of respect. OK, people might respect what someone says, but if you have not been going through that tunnel of darkness of your soul, you cannot really understand someone who is and so you cannot really help him. I think that in this panel you should explore this kind of experiences, because many people get lost in dementia, they are trapped in this nonlinear time. Thank you.

Herrerías: I think it was a very interesting contribution. When I am preparing a clinical homeopathic history, and specifically when the patient gets to the point where he does not know how to explain what is happening to him, that is the moment that he is entering in contact with his deepest internal suffering. I have studied in Mexico, Europe, and Russia, but at present I am following the Indian school. And according to the latest contributions at the vanguard of homeopathy, the way the patient relates his history leads us to understand the basic characteristics of the remedy, of the substance he needs for treatment. That is the moment when I, as homeopath, feel really satisfied, because the patient is really showing me the path, showing me the treatment that is the most similar to his suffering, and therefore it makes it easier for me to understand the needed remedy. So, even though it may seem that you are lost, that you are entering the chaos, what is really happening is that the patient enters the chaos of information where there is no logic any more, no rational thought, because disease, discomfort, is irrational, is energetic at its base, and can only manifest or materialize through physical symptoms. So what you said corresponds to how the unicist classic homeopathy – through the method of vital sensation, or the method of Divya Chhabra, an Indian homeopath – allows us to arrive exactly at the source of the remedy. I do not know if I have answered your question. Is it that prejudice hampers us from getting to the essence?

I think that's it. That's why Hippocrates said to observe the patient and make a diagnosis, and Hahnemann said that the unprejudiced observer – the doctor – can see clearly the deviations from the healthy state of the patient and evaluate what symptoms need to be treated. Thank you.

Audience: I liked what you said a lot, but I want to add what I consider an important point. All these new techniques that are now appearing in the market – for example the work I do, which is healing with symbols and water, or Ho'oponopono, or quantum medicine, or even classic homeopathy – are actually based on the holistic paradigm, so we are working on the basis of waves. Conventional medicine, on the other hand, is based on particles, matter. So we can make experiments based on a mechanistic model and obtain results, but not on the basis of the holistic model, because here we are constantly into new territory, with new conditions. So my point of view is that we do not need to *demonstrate*. What I am experiencing in my daily life with patients is that things are occurring that my small mind is not able to understand. But that I *do not need* to understand either, for me it is sufficient to see results. This is what I wanted to share. Thank you.

Abanades: I'd like to give you the same answer a homeopath gave at the Homeopathic Academy of Barcelona, when I presented scientific evidence of homeopathy. I focused on the subject of the scientific evidence of homeopathy and how can we explain it.

We have a problem, which is that the world we are living in today is mechanist in some respects. Conventional medicine is based on scientific method, and therefore there is a way to make treatments available for patients, through studies, clinical tests, and the like. We can demonstrate what is happening with holistic treatment in various ways. We can simply demonstrate that the quality of life increases in our patients when we give them treatments. It does not matter whether it is a wave or a particle, what matters is that when we apply it the quality of life improves. But it is very important to show what is the scientific base, what mechanisms occur in our body when we apply this therapy or that therapy. Why? Because otherwise we are subject to the risk – and now I am speaking as a homeopathic doctor – that we will be removed from the system and they make us illegal. I do not like to talk from a place of fear, because it is contrary to my religion. I talk from a place of optimism, because I think that truth is truth and will always be. However, if with the rules of this paradigm we do not demonstrate the validity of our therapies, we risk being excluded and some therapies may even vanish. I do not think this will happen because we see new doctors, new therapists, who are perfectly able to study the therapies we apply and find the scientific basis. It is very important to take this into account because there is some risk of exclusion.

Herrerías: I totally disagree. First of all I do not think we are going to be excluded. I have been working with conventional medicine for thirty-five years and with homeopathy for twenty-five. In these twenty-five years I went through various processes and sometimes as a homeopath I did not know what was happening. I knew I was doing things, but I did not completely understand what was happening. Right now I know a bit about homeopathy and I understand how to do a clinical history. I am a doctor, this is the main thing. I wanted to be a doctor since I was three years old. When I arrived at the medical faculty, I got a heavy flu with 40-degree fever and I said: "What am I doing here? The only thing we do is make people get sick."

But with homeopathy I have discovered something new. This morning I was trying to explain Swedenborg. I discovered his writings recently and it helped me understand many things. I recommend it to you if you have not read them. We cannot explain homeopathy from the perspective of another paradigm, so we have to explain it from the paradigm of homeopathy, from our own understanding of what health and disease is. We are talking about correspondences here; we are not talking about the physiological level. There is an edema because there is heart failure, or there is itching because bilirubin is high. This is logical. These are symptoms, they correspond to the diagnostic level of the mechanistic model, which is the model of symptoms. But the disease in its origin is energetic. So we cannot explain homeopathy from a mechanistic paradigm, that does not make any sense. We have to defend this position. I think we are on a journey and that the kind of threats that put the homeopathy at risk of exclusion make no sense. Because we see that patients are improving with homeopathy. I am not talking just about their pathology

I had a patient who had been diagnosed with a brain tumor ten or twelve years earlier. Doctors had tried everything for him, they had given him chemotherapy, radiotherapy. They said he was incurable because he had already had surgery three times. With homeopathy everything changed. In three months there was no tumor, only the scar. But not only that changed, he changed his way of life. That is healing, changing his way to be in life, his way to live in circumstances. And it was not just because he did some sort of coaching (I am not saying that coaching does not work), but because he gained an understanding about how to use and live with his emotions. Once cured, he automatically started to experience what was happening around him in a different way. At that point it no longer made any sense for the tumor to be there, so it disappeared. It disappeared after he changed his way of life. This had nothing to do with reason or mechanistic processes. This is what we are pursuing in classical homeopathy. We want to improve our quality of life, our understanding, our being in life, respecting our environment.

As a doctor, I will take into account the conventional diagnosis, the physical mechanistic diagnosis, but I'll try to treat at the source, which is the energetic imbalance. So I am not going to explain what homeopathy is from a mechanistic paradigm because this does not make any sense and people will never understand us. It's like explaining to a meat-eater that he needs to be vegetarian. It does not make sense. We have to explain using our own paradigm. And our empirical understanding is based on observation, on results, and on reproducibility. This is the most scientific empirical basis, I do not know what can be more scientific than that. In homeopathy we do not work on hypothesis, we work from experience. A hypothesis can be right or wrong. So I do not agree with you.

Dalmau: Well I am in the middle, although I do not think that the two arguments are polar opposites, because in the end we are all saying the same thing. What happens is that there is only one reality. So if you have an objective you want to use all the tools at your disposal so that people can get closer to those therapies.

There are many ways of doing research. Maybe they are not the most adequate for these medical systems, but if today they allow us to arrive at more widespread acceptance I think approximation can be justified. But in any case I am not saying that these methods explain how [homeopathy] works. I do not think that is what Sergio wanted to express.

So today we have some tools that derive from our way of understanding the world. You can use them to understand another way of looking at reality.

Let's talk about acupuncture: today it is finding increasing acceptance, but I do acupuncture and I do not think that it works only because you are stimulating the nervous system – although it does do that. There is also a part that probably has to do with the connective tissue, electromagnetism, and so on. We need to develop the tools. The same happened with classical physics: until well into the last century it saw things in a different way. Then everything changed with quantum physics, which said that the reality was different. Those were the tools they had. Today quantum physics is establishing itself in the scientific field and has made a leap into biology. So we need tools that allow us to understand. The proof is that today, for example, there are ways and methodologies, complete systems, that confirm what you just said: that you cannot study homeopathy from the perspective of biomedicine. You need to devise methods that are in line with the reality of the medical system you are studying. Homeopathy, osteopathy, traditional Tibetan, Chinese medicine, and so on, each has its own reality. You need to find a form that allows you to observe all these realities so that you can maybe find a better understanding of your own reality.

Earlier, we were talking about particles and waves: these are actually one of the bases of quantum physics, the duality. In a real sense there are neither particles nor waves. It all depends on the moment of observation. Einstein already said that mass and energy are exactly the same. So in the end we are talking about the same thing. The only thing is that if I observe the glass from this side I will see the right side, and I will not see the left side. And things are not white or black either, they are white *and* black at same time. Therefore I can get one kind of information with one method and different information with another. I think that probably this can be a way. And at some point in time – although time does not exist, this is another reality – another reality will materialize. Thomas Kuhn, in his theory of scientific revolutions, said it will appear some day. So I do think that all tools are useful and necessary. The question is what is our objective. You can use any tool, they can be useful or not, efficient or not. But the question is: "Where are we going?"

Herrerías: I want to add just one thing. If we limit ourselves too much it is difficult to make progress. The point is to expand our knowledge, our point of view. Within the parameters of the paradigm we are expanding information, and that brings more knowledge. Information cannot be limited just in one way, we always need to increase it, because if quantum physics hadn't done so it would not be at the point where it is now. Progress is always disruptive. To contribute with new ways of envisioning things, of seeing things, and to experiment is always difficult, but we should not be afraid to do it.

Abanades: I thought this was a meeting of integrative medicine, no? Is the topic about integrative medicine or homeopathy? I am a unicist homeopath. I work on patients with my own hands, with subtle energies that God gives us. I can say quite frankly that I do not care what mechanism occurs when I put my hands on a patient. In the framework

of homeopathy I would like to thank all homeopaths and nonhomeo-
path scientists who helped us conduct out studies. So when the government asks us: "What is homeopathy?" we can answer: "Well, we
don't know exactly..." "What are these little globule pills for?" "Well,
we do not know exactly what is inside these globules..." "And if you
go on diluting and diluting, what will you find in the end?" "Well..."

The other day the [TV] channel La Sexta came to our clinic and
asked me two hundred questions about the placebo effect in homeopathy.
I answered as best I could.

But here we are talking about integrative medicine, we really need
to unite, to join forces. Our homeopathy is very good but we must not
forget that conventional medicine is giving us a lot of results and helping us a lot with diagnosis. We really need to unite because if we unite
we will be stronger. If we just stay in our magnificent palaces looking
out at others it could happen – as is already being attempted in some
countries – that homeopathic pharmacies will be shut down. I know
they are excluding many homeopathic remedies simply because we do
not know how to explain what is inside these little globules. And we
cannot allow this to happen. We really need to strengthen our position
because I, for one, very much want to continue giving homeopathy to
my patients. Thank you.

Moderator: I would like to ask the organizers whether we can go on
with a few more questions. I think this discussion has been very con-
structive. We have seen different points of view, legitimate points of
view to which I think we need to respond. Next question, please.

Audience: Hello good afternoon. I am listening with interest. I am a
user of homeopathic medicine. My question is: I tried homeopathy and
it worked, but I am not a scientist. I do not understand what homeopathy does to my body, but I know it works.

Many years ago, when I started with homeopathy the doctor gave
me these globules, these little pills. No pharmacy was selling them at
the time. Today there is actually a critical mass of users of homeop-

athy. I am talking about homeopathy, but I think it is the same with acupuncture, with Tibetan medicine, with Chinese medicine. Users are not stupid: what works, works. We have our criteria. And this critical mass is growing and growing. What can I do about the fact that public health care does not offer any homeopaths or acupuncturists that I can go to? I always need to use a private system. Our governments do not care about our demands. Is it because they are ignorant scientifically talking or is it a political-economic question?

Moderator: Well, this is another question that remains in the air. However, I propose to go back to the main theme: mental health, dementia, Alzheimer's, all those topics that are the reason we are here. And I would like to address a couple of questions to the four speakers that may be closer to what we are discussing. Sometimes it is easier to see things when we go into details instead of getting lost in philosophy. I was very interested in what happens in patients with Alzheimer's or ataxia, for example, when the patient and family realize that something is making the disease accelerate. This worsening usually coincides with a particularly stressful event. In Alzheimer's often the patient experiences a loss of self esteem, or feels he is a burden for the family, or simply experiences a stressful event that acts as a trigger of the disease.

Here again we are not talking about particles, but information, meaning. It is more difficult to talk about molecules or an alteration of neurotransmitters that surely accompany such an event at an organic level, but the trigger for such an event has to do with emotions, with experience, with living. In neuropsychiatric pathology, I think this is a very important point both for recognizing what has caused the disease to develop and for the treatment. I would like the speakers, or someone from the audience, give their opinion.

So the question is: are we starting from the assumption that our brain and mental diseases are in resonance with our experiences, with our emotions, and also with our beliefs? Because it is not what happens to us that matters, it is how we live the experience. The patient Teresa told us about this morning was not in so much misery – the daughter confirmed that – but she was *living* this way. That has such a huge importance in neuropsychiatric pathology and particularly in dementia, and it is worth researching and paying attention to from the point of view of the treatment, regardless what kind of treatment you choose. This opens a broad topic: energetic psychology techniques and so on. Maybe we have not enough time for that, but I would like to pose at least one last question to Dr. Phuntsog Wangmo.

You said that is better not to reach to the point of treatment, that the ideal is prevention. I would like to ask you how can we anticipate, how can we relieve those poisons that are part of us or that as you have said we all have on some level? But then we also have the contemporary scientific theories about the stress response, the relaxation response, the authentic technology of the consciousness, which is meditation, the many things we can do in a state of apparent health. I do not think that anybody is really healthy. Can you give us your thoughts on what we can do for prevention? This would be especially relevant for people who want to help, therapists and caregivers.

Wangmo: Thank you. It has been very interesting to listen to all of you.

There are several things we can do toward the prevention of serious mental diseases. Both physically and mentally. And also environmental.

In terms of the physical factors, as I have said before, we are living with or we are composed of the five elements and both an excess or a deficiency is negative. To avoid excesses [and deficiencies] first of all you need to know what your personality is and what category you belong to. But basically you should eat more cooked food and especially drink hot water.

The earth and water element are heavy and water is cold and heavy. So our body needs digestive heat, that is very important. The stomach is like the field we are cultivating and for the field heat is important. You all know that even if we cultivate a simple plant the plant needs a certain temperature. Heat alone is not enough to make it grow, but it is fundamental. Everything we eat needs to be digested and then regenerated. The body cells need digestive heat in order to regenerate substances. So for prevention heat is especially important. For example, if you eat raw, heavy, and uncooked food this can easily kill heat. A simple thing is to drink hot water, or hot water with honey. Honey is sweet, but its nature is light, warm, and rough. The light part of the honey has the potential to break down fat and has the energy to make circulate whatever needs to circulate in the body. The rough part melts the fatty or the condensed heavy part. This is one of the most important ways to prevent Alzheimer's, mental diseases, dementia, and depression.

Mentally, whatever happens to you try to keep a positive outlook. For example, if you have a serious disease, try to think of it as a good opportunity: if it is related to your past karma, it is an opportunity to clean it. Or you could think that scientists can use your body to create a new treatment for other patients. So try to be positive, no matter what happens in life. I think these are methods to avoid mental diseases.

Moderator: Thank you. We will finish this session here. I would like to thank Dr. Herrerías, Dr. Dalmau, Dr. Wangmo, and Dr. Abanades for generously sharing their knowledge and all of you for your presence here and your attention. Thank you so much everyone.

Dementia

Moderator: Dr. Carmen Martínez

Ms. Neus Rodríguez is founder and president of the Fundació Uszheimer, an organization dedicated to helping people affected by neuro-degenerative diseases such as Alzheimer's. She is also the sponsor of the foundation and the director of the Uszheimer interdisciplinary group. Its primary objectives are to delay the degenerative process of these diseases through psychosocial stimulation; to improve cognitive, functional, and social performance; and to offer support and guidance to the families of those affected.

Given the biopsychosocial impact caused by neurodegenerative diseases in our society, the Fundació Uszheimer focuses its efforts on three areas: social work; education; and social and medical research in the field of neurodegenerative diseases.

PRESENTATION

NEUS RODRÍGUEZ
Psychosocial Intervention in Dementia:
The Uszheimer Program
Documentary on Alzheimer's Disease,
Winner of the 2013 Solé Tura Awards

I would like to thank the organizers of the event, of this symposium, for giving me the opportunity to understand a little better these different types of medicine, this possibility of having different ways to intervene in disease. I really think that I have a broader vision now. Just to give you an introduction, I think that all of us here share something: we see the patient as a whole. We do not see patients from the point of view of the diseases afflicting them. We really see the human being as a whole system, with everything it includes in its vastness. I also think that this is certainly not an easy journey and it is difficult for conventional medicine to recognize these interventions, but it is not at all impossible. In fact twenty years ago when we started our path, our journey was focused on raising the awareness that the people who suffer from Alzheimer's need specific treatment. I went everywhere, throughout Spain and Cuba. I spoke at universities, trying to communicate what we wanted to do, what our mode of intervention is. I attempted to communicate that we had achieved important results. I think that if you are persistent and professional, in the end you will be rewarded. And this applies to everything. Nothing happens overnight. Here in our country alternative or nonconventional medicine is not recognized, but we have the long and difficult job of making it known. We need to raise awareness, to try to transmit information, train the professionals, but also communicate with the people on the streets. This is very important. This is just an introduction, just to start my talk. I want to thank the organizers and also everyone who has participated, because everyone has contributed to widening my point of view.

Our foundation was born twenty years ago when we wanted to have a broad approach for assisting people who suffer from Alzheimer's. It focuses its efforts on three operative areas: social work, teaching, and intervention. These three approaches basically enable us to see each patient as a whole system, as I mentioned before, including everything around them.

Social Work

The social or charity program aims at facilitating the access to stimulation therapy for those affected by cognitive deterioration and, as consequence, present a moderate grade of dependence. It also offers some resources to satisfy other issues that could come about in the process of neurodegenerative disease, such as isolation, family accompanying, economic subsidies, and psychotherapy.

What does our institution do? First of all, when a patient comes to us, we carry out a diagnosis of the disease. We already have a diagnosis, because they have been diagnosed by a neurologist, but what we want to know is, within the pathology, what part is mostly affected: is it the attention, or the concentration, or the immediate memory, for example. So, after a battery of tests, we know what kind of intervention we are going to apply. It will be an individualized treatment, specific for that very patient.

Teaching

Within this line of intervention we focus on giving specific training to the professionals involved, meaning everyone working with this kind of patient in elder homes, day care centers, and sociomedical programs, including big hospitals. We aim to teach them what they should do, how things should be done, what attitude they should have when confronting the behavior of the patients. This sort of approach is not something new today, now people can get information from social media, from the Internet, but twenty years ago we did not have this information at all. So we used to see patients in the emergency rooms of big hospitals tied to beds with security belts because they wanted to jump off or go away. We saw that education and training of professionals was necessary. It was obvious that we needed to raise the awareness of the need for a different approach: for example, letting relatives hold the hands of the patients while they were in the emergency room helped very much if they had to undergo medical examination. These patients needed to be treated, needed to undergo tests, but they needed to be with relatives in order to be relieved from their anguish. In fact they could not recognize voices, they could not recognize what they were being asked. Very often in big hospitals you would hear doctors asking "Do you know who you are? Do you know where you are now?" and this created more anguish in them, they really wanted to get out and ended up tied to the hospital beds. It was very important to raise the awareness of the professionals.

Research

We also work on research. In this area, we have agreements with the universities of Barcelona (for example with Ramon Llull University, with the University of Barcelona, and with the Autonomous University of Barcelona), also for other subjects, like physiotherapy. When interns come to our foundation, I like to read what they write, I like to know what they think and hear their opinion, because sometimes they can see things that we cannot really detect in terms of treatment. So, what foundation's aim with these teaching agreements is to provide some tools to those who have a degree in psychology, social assistance, and social education to enable them to treat professionally and accurately. Twenty years ago, when a psychologist would come to our foundation and had to change a patient's diaper, he would say: "I'm working toward a degree!" I would say: "You will never know an Alzheimer's patient if you do not go into the toilet with him and see how he looks at the mirror, how he talks to the mirror, and all those kinds of details." This is just a little example to tell you how we want the patient to really be seen and treated from every point of view. All the people our institution works with not only have a degree and understand what the project is about, but also have a personality able to understand the feelings and emotions of the patients. So the profile of the people who work in our institution is not based on professional qualifications alone: they also have to be connected to their own emotions, be open minded, and really love their job and especially the patient. This is something that you acquire only when you work with these patients on a daily basis.

Primary Objectives

Our objective, then, is to offer treatment based on global cognitive stimulation. The word "global" was not very widespread twenty years ago. People did not understand that you have to consider the global field affected by the disease, because Alzheimer's affects not just the patient, but the patient's entire social environment as well. For example, if we have an Alzheimer's patient in a family, the social environment changes, all of it. There is a time *before* and a time *after* this event. When a family member comes to me at the foundation and says a relative was diagnosed one week before, I tell him or her that he had been suffering from it for many years already. And when they think about they realize that it is true: they could see some signs already three or four years ago. Why is that? Because when the memory loss starts, normally these patients try to hide it from the family, they think it's something sort of normal because they are getting older. This means that diagnosis is delayed, which is bad because the sooner we can diagnose, the sooner we treat. Usually when the family realizes that deterioration has taken place it is because the patient has done something major and striking that made them aware of it. But there was something also *before*, for example social isolation. The patient did not want to go where he used to go, he did not want to interact with people he normally interacted with because he did not want people to realize that he was suffering of this. So often relatives think that they are suffering from depression because they isolate themselves in a circle where they feel quiet and safe.

Yesterday Dr. Teresa Herrerías was speaking about how scared an Alzheimer's patient was. All Alzheimer's patients have fear. They are terribly frightened of all the information they receive because they cannot process it in the way we do and this causes painful anguish. If somebody were to ask me what an Alzheimer's patients actually feels, what are the symptoms, based on my personal experience I would always say that the symptom is fear. Fear twenty-four hours a day. This is often expressed through anxiety, compulsory eating, walking up and down. Maybe I am a little off topic, but I really think it is important to transmit the knowledge we have acquired in the course of the past twenty years. And this is what we see every day.

What do we do in our program? We try to reduce the level of dependence that is the result of any neurodegenerative disease. How? We try to keep the patients active the whole day through a series of stimulations so that the family members also can be free during these hours. But it's not just about giving the relatives a break for a few hours; I always try to make this clear to the family members when they come to me. We are helping the Alzheimer's patients. On top of that, if the relatives can be free for a couple of hours and go on with their lives with less dependence on the part of the patient, it is better for them. But what must be clear is that the patient can be helped. We can do a series of therapies that will allow them to live better with their disease and improve the quality of their life. We know that Alzheimer's patients tend to isolate themselves. We try to work on this, on the social aspect, we try to make them interact. We have had patients who actually fell in love while they were in our foundation. Everything is possible, even love between two patients. When one of them died, the woman kept an empty chair at her side and was always asking: "Where is he?" She could not really express her feelings through words, because she did not have sufficient vocabulary, but she was feeling that her companion was missing. This is just an anecdote, one of the many from the last twenty years.

Sustaining the Patient's Environment Throughout the Process of Illness

We not only attend to the patient, we also take care of the family members, of the social environment around the patient, and of all the problems that are brought about by the disease. We know that the disease can last a very long time, up to sixteen years, if the patients are physically well and are not suffering from other pathologies due to their age. And in this period many situations may occur, like the death of a son or the illness of some loved ones. So we also help the family members by advising them how to manage the whole situation. We have to work together, together for the well-being of the patient. This is very clear for the institution: the priority is always the patient. And then the family. The more the family understands how to treat the patient, how to understand the disease, how to behave when specific circumstances occur, the more the patient will experience an improvement in his quality of life. Because the environment will be more peaceful, the family members will see the disease in a different way if they have more information, if they have more resources at their disposal. That is why we have created support groups. Support groups are not just groups where everybody can express their feelings: they are guided by professionals with a specific objective and specific strategies for each meeting, so that people can have a sort of training and know what to expect during the disease.

We also have a program for orientation and training for the family members, I already spoke about that a little. It's a service for every family; they can come any time to see us and talk to the professionals because we are always with them. The professionals working with us know perfectly well how to behave toward every patient, because they spend many hours with them.

Within the stimulation therapy program I was telling you about, we do not just work on the cognitive skills through memory workshops, we also work on psychomotricity. Twenty years ago, when a poster on psychomotricity was presented at a conference, it seemed something almost esoteric that a physiotherapist would do exercises with an Alzheimer's patient. But it has been demonstrated that physiotherapy is also very important. It is not just passive gymnastics, or a way to reinforce muscles, it is very important to coordinate movements and work on many areas of the patient's body so that he or she can keep walking and do many other movements.

Stimulation can also occur through arts. Twenty years ago while we were presenting an exhibition of paintings at a congress, Dr. Martinez Lage of the University of Navarra told me: "Neus, the art therapy you are doing is very important, much more important than you think." We have developed a special technique for the patients. They are not just painting a little landscape or a duck that we show them. It is more than that, it is a technique, a way of painting with them. Downstairs in the reception we have a book on art therapy that we can send to you all for free. If you go to our website you can see it, it is a manual in Spanish on cognitive stimulation. [The title is *Manual de intervención en demencias*.] We published it together with the European Community and the Ministry of Social Affairs. We did it for free, but on condition that it be provided for free to all the institutions that work with Alzheimer's patients.

So, after twenty years I can tell you that art therapy is really useful, as that doctor said. Our work does not have an empirical basis; this is something a little subjective. But in these patients the right hemisphere works much better than the left one. We do not have an academic publication, even though we have worked seriously on it together with many psychologists, pedagogues, and educators. However, you can see that all of these areas are very well structured: we have art therapy, music therapy, reminiscence, mime, tales and legends, and dance therapy. We already have a didactic unit that works on how to structure and validate the programs in this manual. So, we have worked very much, but I would like to do more, because it has not yet been demonstrated scientifically. In these patients the right hemisphere, which has to do with creativity, works much better. Many patients have never painted, most of them never picked up a brush in their whole life. When giving art therapy courses in Spain I was telling the professionals working with me that I needed people who had never painted in their life because they follow the guidelines we give for this technique more accurately.

Home Service

Why do we offer this service? Because as the physical deterioration of some of our patients increased, they did not want us to give up the stimulation therapy we provided for them. But at the same time they could not be moved from home. They already had a reduced mobility, so it was a problem to take them from one part of Barcelona to another. So we created a program for stimulation therapy at home for the Alzheimer's patients and others affected by neurodegenerative illness. The provincial administration of Huelva supported us. Eleven professionals from our institution went to the Huelva mountains and trained eleven professionals to be able to give this kind of home service. So we provide the same stimulation therapy that we offer at our center in the patient's home. What's more, we also train the family members. This provides additional support.

In Barcelona, we also had the support of the provincial administration and we carried out this training for three years in the municipality of Castelldefels with wonderful results. The municipality is really happy with this service, because we are not just washing the patients but we are stimulating them, working with them and their family.

In this slide you can see the support group for the families, we already explained that. We try to encourage dialogue to exchange experiences and to also provide training.

Social Assistance Program

We have a social assistance program as well. Twenty years ago we did not have the Dependency Law[3] in Barcelona. Old people were coming and saying: "You are asking 400 euros, I have no money to do this kind of treatment." Now we have agreements with the regional government on the basis of the Dependency Law, so the foundation does not have to leave anyone knocking at its door without help.

Awareness Program

Five years ago we established the Solé Tura Award as part of our awareness program. I say five years because the first year we presented this award to public and private institutions. Jordi Solé Tura was a part of our foundation, it was a great honor for us. When he died, together with his family we wanted to make this form of assistance permanent and use the name of this well-known person for the award in order to work on raising awareness. The general objective was to try to show this reality to many people. We created the award so that short filmmakers could present their work. And we worked with two motivations: to give cinematography students a chance to present their work and gain an award and to raise awareness of neurodegenerative disease through these short films. The first year we did staged the event at the Picasso Museum in Barcelona, the second year in the La Pedrera building in Paseo de Gracia, and the third year in the Agbar tower. This year we did it at the Biomedical Research Park in Barcelona. This event focuses on the presentation of films on people with

---

3   A law passed in 2006 with the objective of improving the quality of life of individuals in a situation of dependency, due to disability, illness, or advanced age, and alleviating the financial and time burden on their relatives.

neurodegenerative diseases. This year we expanded the topic to include other diseases such as bipolar disorder and stroke. And this gives us a lot of material. So when we try to raise awareness in different neighborhoods, we show these movies. Sometimes an image has much more impact than words.

Sharing Memories

This is a program we have developed with the educational consortium of Catalonia in order to work with children so that they understand at an early age the impact of this disease. We do not teach them about pathology, but about what this disease implies. From school age they learn that they do not have to fear a grandparent who does not call them by name or recognize them, for example. They have to understand the behavior of these patients. This is a program we carry out at various schools in Barcelona. We give talks in the schools, and then they come to visit us at the foundation and share some projects with the elderly. Each box like this, for example, contains things that represent memories Alzheimer's patients shared with children who interviewed them. And then when the children give the box to the patients it is very emotional because some patients are able to recognize inside this box things about their own history. So it allows these children to better understand things, and sometimes they are surprised by what they learn. One of the patients was a Barcelona football club supporter whose membership number was eight, and some of the children thought it was just amazing to have contact with someone with such an ancient membership number.

We offer an innovative school model based on the application of different fields of knowledge, such as neuropsychology, nursing, pedagogy, social education, physiotherapy, fine arts, and performing arts. Professionals from all different fields form an interdisciplinary team. Not multidisciplinary, but interdisciplinary. Why? Because they work together, it is not like some of them work this way and some others work that way. They work in an interconnected way. For example, if we have a physiotherapy activity the psychologist is also there. We work in an interdisciplinary way, we all share the same objective. Specific objectives are to motivate and find new ways to use the theoretical and practical knowledge of our professionals. Why? Because if I am a nurse and listen to the language of my psychologist colleague this allows me to learn from him but he is also learning things from me. So we will all be working and learning at the same time, thus broadening our knowledge. All of us work and learn at the same time.

We also teach our interns, our undergraduates, what we do. The objective is that at the end of their internship they are able to say: "I have really learned what an Alzheimer's patient is."

And we give therapeutic instruments and tools to families.

Activities

We also offer training courses and workshops. We travel throughout Spain. Sometimes we are invited to explain our activities, and we are always open, because people need to know about what we do. This does not mean it is just perfect. We learn a lot of things every time we prepare a course or a conference: we have to review our daily work, to try to improve every day, and to learn from others and from other communities. We have learned so much visiting other communities.

We also participate in conferences, seminars, trainings, courses, and conventions with universities, as I already mentioned. We work really closely with public institutions. For example, every time the regional government asks us to participate in a conference or in debate, we always go so that more people can learn from our experience. And we have also collaborated with the municipalities. As an entity, we are governed by the Barcelona municipality and the provincial administration of Barcelona. We are also under the Board of Health. We try to always work hand in hand with the institutions. I think that is the place where we should be. Since they have no money, they do not pay us, they leave us alone. But of course we try to get their support for what we do.

Research

Why research? Because we are always open to help. For example, when an undergraduate from university is doing a research project about emotional support or about pathologies of caregivers, we are always open to help.

Sorry, I do not like to read from slides – I would rather talk from my experience and from my heart. Current research topics include memory units and fibromyalgia. Fibromyalgia patients also suffer from memory losses. We have been working with a related association in the area of cognitive stimulation for these patients.

"Help us not to forget" is the motto of our foundation. Not to forget history, not to forget about them, not to forget their lives.

Everything that was presented here these past few days was so interesting to me. So I took good notes in order to further widen our work with Alzheimer's patients. And I would like to tell you that they are all very special in their situations. You see them in these pictures, all of them suffer from Alzheimer's, but each of them is very special. I cannot look at them, sorry [emotional pause]. I have learned to love them so much, and they are really special. When you really get to know them, when you communicate with them, you learn to love them so much.

Now I am going to show you the film that won the second prize in this year's Solé Tura Award, the awareness program I told you about earlier. Before the Dr. Martí's talk, I want you to see this film, so that you can get a better view of the situation and can better understand this kind of patients. You have so much to contribute from your disciplines, you have so much to offer us from your expertise. So, please, now watch the film. *[Ten-minute screening of documentary in Spanish.]*

Can you see in this film the love this patient has around her? It really helps her to go on. But you see also the suffering of this relative, you have seen him burst into tears. Losing your life is so cruel. I have seen many people dying from different pathologies, but to lose the history of your life is so cruel. To lose your history. Only love remains, and the love around this patient will help her to better live to the end of her life.

(2nd session)

Dr. Guillem Martí has been coordinator of the Psychology Department of the Fundació Uszheimer since 2004. He holds a degree in psychology from the University of Barcelona (2003), a certificate in education skills in psychology (May 2004), and a master's degree in neuroscience and neuropsychology from the IAEU (Instituto de Altos Estudios Universitarios) program at the University of Barcelona (2007).

Dr. Martí also participated in the Catalan Neuropsychology Society Conference (2005, Barcelona); in the National Alzheimer's Disease Congress (2005, Murcia); and in the Recent Developments in the Multidisciplinary Approach to Psychogeriatric Behavior Disorders (2006, Barcelona).

PRESENTATION

GUILLEM MARTÍ
Dementia Spectrum: Dealing with the Ill Person

Good morning. I am Guillem Martí. First of all, I want to thank the organizers for having asked me here. After this emotional film I'll try to talk about the approach of families to dementia, how they react to the hard blow of knowing they have at home a patient affected by dementia, and how the main caregiver or the family members manage their emotions.

First of all, there is the diagnosis of the disease. As you well know we have different kinds of medicine, different points of view, different perspectives, but detection and diagnosis in our foundation start with little things detected by families: for example that the individual is doing strange things, forgets little things, forgets the keys; this can be the trigger of a request for a new type of help, from a professional, they want to know what's happening to their relative. So, we start here: this has an impact on the family and is causing crisis in this family. I'll explain how we can manage this crisis in an interdisciplinary approach. With this kind of disease, a diagnosis cannot be made by only one professional, by only one psychologist or neurologist or doctor. It has to be an interdisciplinary diagnosis, where each professional contributes something. Each of them has to offer their own grain of salt and say "this patient has this disease."

But what is the objective of a diagnosis? In the end, the objective is not only to give a label, and say "this person has Alzheimer's" or "this person has vascular dementia." The objective is to interpret and understand what are the needs of these patients in order for them to have a better life. As Neus explained, we have interns in our foundation and I always tell the psychology students that simply spending many hours in an office making diagnoses, applying some clinical trial batteries is absolutely useless if it doesn't make the patient feel better, if it doesn't mean a better quality of life for the patient. Everything has to have an objective, and this is our objective as professionals.

But what happens when the family receives this diagnosis? Each family is different, of course, each family has specific features, and every caregiver feels it in a different way. So, the understanding of a disease like Alzheimer's depends on different things. For example, is the family open to change? Are they willing to reorganize their daily functioning? How has the family lived in the past, what is the relationship between parents and children, between the patient and his or her partner, what is the history behind the patient? What about the family structure, the culture, the emotional culture? Sometimes elderly people come from a culture where feelings are a little bit something to hide. And this makes it difficult for the main caregiver to implement all these changes and to accept the disease that has come to the family. We cannot forget the socioeconomic level. As you know, treating this disease costs a lot of money, we need a lot of resources to take care of these kind of patients. Families have to understand these facts and learn to work with the situation.

The first step in this process of managing is for the family to visit our foundation, or their doctor, or a neurologist, and ask: "How do we cope with this? How can we live with our relative's disease? How can we manage all the problems that will arise?" So the first person they find is the professional who sees the family. As professionals we have to help them define the problems caused by dementia at home. For example, we look at the daily activities of the patient, the history of the family, and life of this patient, then we make the caregiver or the relative understand what the word dementia entails, what we may have to face. Of course, we do not have to talk about the future when we first see this family. I might say to them: "Let's think about today. We don't have to worry about what will happen in six, seven, or eight years, we'll face it when it comes." Of course, it depends very much on the moment when the family comes to the institution, an early stage is not the same as a late stage The stage of the disease is very important. Needs will change for the caregiver in each stage of the disease.

And then when there is a diagnosis the family has to decide what to do: should they have the patient admitted to a residential center so they can forget about this daily burden? Keeping the patient at home is not only an objective burden, involving physical work and expenses, but also a subjective burden with stress, anxiety and burn out for the main caregiver. Plus there are all the problems surrounding patients with Alzheimer's or other dementias. If the family as a whole decides not to have the patient admitted to a nursing facility or center, do they need help at home? If they ask for help, we also have other resources: we have day care centers, professional caregivers coming to their home, homeworkers, and even, when they are in a very late stage, a day hospital. Our foundation has a day care center, and Neus already explained our work.

When we receive these families in our institution, if they are in an early stage they lack information. So we have a role of guiding, which does not mean making decisions. For example, I have a recent case where the brother of a patient died. If the family asks: "What should we do? Do we have to tell the patient or not?" I am not going to make this decision, but I will be able, maybe, to guide them, to council them, making them understand what is better for the patient. Is this going to be useful for the patient? Let us think about pros and cons. It's the family that has to make the final decision, never the professionals, that is not our role.

We have three stages in the assistance of families. We have this lack of information, the exhaustion in the intermediate stage, then the overwhelming grief. We have seen the case of that man, the main caregiver in the film. He is starting to enter the final stage. He is not only tired, he is a little overwhelmed, it's a situation beyond his capacity. Maybe he has understood that he prefers to keep his loved one at home, despite all the physical, economical and emotional costs it entails. OK, he has weighed the pros and cons and has made this decision to keep her at home.

The first stage is lack of information. When a family comes to us and asks: "What is that our relative has? What is dementia? What is Alzheimer's? What is Parkinson's? What is this Lewy body dementia?" we have to try to help them, inform them that the patient has this kind of cognitive deterioration, that the emotional field is also affected; we tell them about depression symptoms, mainly in early stages of Alzheimer's, that are not always present but that most patients have. So, this assistance, providing information in the early stage, has to help the caregiver, the family, to make decisions and consequently make some agreements with the patient. Because in the early stages the patient still has some capacities, and is still able to make decisions; so at that moment, the family has to negotiate with him or her, to make an agreement. "What do we do? Do you want to go to the center to do stimulation therapy?" Sometimes families tell us that he or she does not want to come. Maybe in this family the patient has not yet authorized others to make decisions on his behalf. These things occur in the first stages, and we, as professionals, have to try to support the caregiver, and to monitor how the caregiver is experiencing this first stage: how he feels, and how he understands that the disease is affecting the house or the family.

In the intermediate stage what families and caregivers need is information, training, and guidance. They might participate in courses, learn how to manage the emotional burden, learn self-control techniques. Most of all, they have to learn how to prevent depression, for example. Later we will talk about the impact of this disease on the caregivers and how we manage emotions. But as Neus told you before, in our foundation we have support groups for families. That is very important. Of course, we do not give them therapy, but we share experiences. Maybe some caregivers have more experience, and are able to support others who are just beginning to live this role. So they can share techniques, and little everyday strategies may be really useful. Sometimes in these first periods they are disoriented and overwhelmed because they receive so much information, and simple advice from people who have more experience may help a lot for someone who is just beginning the process.

This is why these support groups are really important. And most of all, in these initial and intermediate stages the emotional burden of caring for a patient at home has to be evaluated; that is very important. So the families that need information and do not come to a center like ours, where do they go? The professionals who get this kind of question are usually general practitioners; families tend to go to them for day-to-day needs. And maybe this is a result of the way primary care is handled today. Here in Barcelona, for example, it is difficult sometimes to get consultations with a specialist, like a neurologist for instance, as often as needed. So general practitioners end up having to deal with those issues and have to be trained in this area.

And then in the final stage of the disease, after eight or nine years of evolution, we see other types of issues. Sometimes, as professionals, we are not very prepared, and it's important to have some training in these areas. Last year in our institution we had the relative of a patient who was a lawyer and had spent his whole life making powers of attorney, living wills, and so on, and he explained to us the legal problems that relatives and caregivers might encounter if they don't take care of the legal aspects as well. Sometimes families ask questions about legal things, and even if we, the professionals, do not know the answer in every case, anyway we can guide them. At most we can say, "You should ask this or that type of professional, you might go to Social Services," and so on. Sometimes on the level of primary care doctors have not this kind of information, possibly due to a lack of time for training, and additionally because consultations are very short. So families ask us for this kind of information and sometimes we have to try to raise awareness. Personally speaking, I had a chance to work in an interdisciplinary team, and I really learned a lot from the other professionals in the team, like the social educator or the social worker, for instance. But sometimes primary care doctors do not have this chance and all this information is beyond their training. So we have to give this kind of guidance to the families when they ask for it.

In terms of social work tasks we have to perform for caregivers, all health care professionals – doctors, nurses, psychologists, community workers, social workers, and family workers – have to be able to evaluate and treat possible pathologies, continually assess the caregiver (not the patient), give him/her health care training, detect possible complications, and most of all, one of the most important points, prevent burnout. When the caregiver of a patient in a late stage burns out, what do we have to do with this patient? Often the family throws in the towel, because the late stage can be so overwhelming that it goes beyond the capacity of the caregiver or family. And when the emotional and physical burden is so heavy, caregivers begin to neglect themselves. We have to prevent this sort of burnout because it has an impact on the main caregiver, who puts himself or herself at risk of suffering from other diseases as a consequence. We see this every day as professionals. For example, family members come to us and say: "I can't stand it anymore." Why? Because you are feeling bad physically or emotionally? Because your family is not helping you? Let us look at your family history, your children, brothers and sisters-in-law: are they helping or not?

In the case in the film, it seems like the caregiver had some kind of professional help. But he was coping with the main daily activities, he was the main caregiver, and that mere fact put him in a position of risk. Which kind of options do we have? We can offer support groups, mutual help groups, family associations, and family therapy, if needed.

So to conclude the first part of my talk we can say that the family is the main resource for the patient. If a patient has no family, surely the management of the disease is going to be lacking, things will be deficient. We have to consider what close relationships the patient has. Sometimes we have seen couples that lived together, their relationship was not good, and now one of them is suffering from this disease, and the other one ends up at home with the patient. "What do I have to do?"

that person might say. "We don't have a good relationship." We have to face these situations as professionals. But as I said before it is very important that we never make decisions. In our institution we offer guidance, but we do not make decisions. We have to help people make the best decisions so that both they and the patient can have the best possible quality of life. That is essential thing for us as professionals – in my case as a psychologist: we have the same objective, the quality of life of the patients has to be the best possible.

We also have to put limits on our involvement as professionals. That is why, as we have seen before, we need to coordinate well with other professionals working in the field. This way we can provide the best possible care.

Now that I have explained all the stages following the diagnosis, we should examine the impact of the disease on a caregiver. I am going to be quicker, because we do not have time anymore.

What are the factors that increase the burden? We have conducted a lot of research on that issue; the conclusions do not always coincide, but all of the studies describe many risk factors that can result in this overburden for the caregiver. We can differentiate between factors having to do with the patient and factors having to do with the caregiver.

Let us consider the burdening factors coming from the patient. We can have a very serious, very intense dementia, which is obviously quite different from when we have a very light dementia. If we have a case of Alzheimer's that develops in four years it is not the same as a case that has been going on for thirteen or fourteen years. The burden is very different. Then we have the specific symptoms of the disease: we can have hallucinations, delusions, confusions, aggressiveness, agitation. All of this results in a burden for the caregiver, but this obviously has to do with the patient.

Then we have factors that have to do with the caregiver. Sometimes the person taking on this role is already older, sometimes is the partner of the patient, of the same age. The caregiver's physical health might not be so good, with the pathologies of old age. He or she could also have a prior history of depression. In a situation like this we will have a recurrence of depression, and the caregiver will not be able to take care of the patient in the best possible way. Sometimes the caregiver does not really understand what the disease is and what kind of care is necessary, and that creates more burden. It's more tiring to do something when you don't understand the type of patient you are caring for. And then there is the issue of managing the psychiatric manifestations of the disease in the patient. With all of that, the family members of Alzheimer's patients who are the main caregivers are more at risk of other diseases than other caregivers who are not the main ones. That means there is a special focus on the main caregiver, who much more than the others can be at risk of diseases such as osteomuscular disorders and other pain symptoms, cardiovascular diseases, gastrointestinal disorders, immunological diseases, respiratory problems. Caregivers can be affected by physical disorders because they fail to take care of themselves. They have no free time anymore. They don't go to the doctor because they have to take care of the patient. Sometimes family members tell me: " I can't take it anymore." And I ask: "But are you taking care of yourself as a person, as a caregiver?" Most of the time they say: "No, I have no time. I can't go to the doctor, I feel pain here, I have headaches." But they do not treat these issues, they just put it aside, because the family member who is sick is the most important person.

According to some studies, among the caregivers of Alzheimer's patients 54% are affected by anxiety, 28% have depression, and 17% are hypochondriac. So as a result of all of these manifestations of dementia, of Alzheimer's disease, the caregivers basically stop taking care of themselves. If the caregivers do not take care of themselves, they cannot take care of other people in an adequate way. This is what we try to explain to the families: if we want to be able to take care of other people we need to be healthy and we need to take care of ourselves.

To conclude, I would like to briefly talk about the behavior that we need to adopt as relatives or caregivers in order to manage all the problems we find in patients with Alzheimer's or dementia. Physical contact is important; we need to be able to manage emotions. We need to try to understand why such situations are occurring. And we need to find a framework in order to classify and understand that everything the patient is going through is caused by a disease. We cannot just hold the patient guilty, like some relatives sometimes do. As a family member we cannot simply assign blame to the patient. If we make an effort to understand what the patient is going through, we will be able to provide and take care, and we will be able to manage both the emotional and physical burden.

I could not really say everything I wanted to say, but unfortunately we no longer have any time. I would like to thank you for the attention both for me and for Neus. And thank you again for inviting us.

(3rd session)

Dr. Rakdo Lobsang Tenzin Rinpoche is a Tibetan doctor and researcher. He trained under several important academics in Tibetan medicine, including Toru Tsenam Rinpoche and Lobsang Wangchuck. Between 1983 and 1985, his work focused on the research and publication of rare Tibetan texts on medicine, history, and Buddhism. For one year, he worked as editor of the publication *Tibetan People* in the autonomous region of Tibet.

A year later, he exiled to India and worked as a professor at the Tibetan Medical and Astrological Institute in Dharamsala. This was a period of intense activity for him, during which he dedicated himself to the teaching of Tibetan medicine, as well as linguistics, astrology and Buddhist philosophy.

Between 1993 and 1996, he taught at the Tibetan Medicine Department of the Central Institute of Higher Tibetan Studies (CIHTS) in Sarnath. He currently teaches, practices medicine, and researches at the CIHTS medical clinic. His extensive research work has led to the creation of over 100 different medicines.

PRESENTATION

LOBSANG TENZIN
The Traditional Tibetan Medicine Approach to the Western Concept of Dementia

Thank you. It is a great pleasure to attend this conference. I have learned a lot from the previous speakers and their inspiring presentations.

Before I go into my topic I would like to spend a few minutes sharing with you information about our situation in India, which is where I live. Before 2010 Tibetan medicine was not recognized by the Indian government. Back in 2008 a group of scholars of Tibetan and also Hindi medicine formed a special team to pursue governmental recognition of Tibetan medicine, and by 2010 the government recognized it as an independent medicine. So now we are developing and practicing Tibetan medicine well in India. That does not mean that now the work is finished; there is much more to do, we need to develop it in every area. I work at the Central University of Tibetan Studies, a university founded by the Indian government where we can study all five of the major sciences. So far we have over 400 students, 60 faculties, and about 50 administrators. We have not only Tibetan students but also international students, research students, undergraduate students, and a program of graduate studies. We also have PhD students: they study for two years, get a diploma, and then leave.

Thank you for listening to this, I just wanted to use this opportunity to share with you the situation of Tibetan medicine in India. Now I will go on to my topic.

I previously prepared a PowerPoint presentation, but this morning somehow the technology does not work, so I hope I will not make you bored. I don't want to explain a lot about the basis of Tibetan medicine, but if I don't explain it at all there is no way to start. So I will explain it just a little.

Firstly let's look at the definition of disease. I am not sure if there is an exact equivalent in English, but in Tibetan we use the term *ned* [both for conditions of disorder and the humors]. The body is composed of five elements and three humors. If there is any alteration in these, it will change the body and mind mechanisms and cause suffering either physically or mentally.

In general, during the time of the formation of the body and its functions and during life, for survival, everything is based on the three *ned* or *duwa*. If the three *ned* undergo any alteration then we have suffering. Why do they change? They are changed by certain conditions. In Tibetan medicine we never suppose that the *ned* or disease comes from outside to the inside. What we think is that we already have the seed of the disease or *ned* in our body, so once we have a secondary condition illness manifests. This is *ned*.

Someone explained the cause of disease yesterday, so I don't want repeat that. At this moment our main topic is the *ned* of mental illnesses. As we said before, there are three direct or primary causes of illness. Among these three the cause of mental disease is a disturbance of the *lung* or wind element. What is the cause of a *lung* disorder? Yesterday we explained the three poisons. Among these, attachment is the cause or condition of an air imbalance, a *lung* disorder. There are many ways of explaining attachment. There is a more rough level of attachment: for example if we see a nice flower or a nice object and we want to have it, that is a rough, material attachment. But there is also a more subtle level of attachment. I am not going to explain all kinds of attachment, how they happen and so forth; there is not enough time.

But why do we have attachment? What is its cause? It is because of ignorance. We have dualistic vision so we believe that objects exist, we do not know that everything is empty. This is called *marigpa* or ignorance. There are many different levels of ignorance. Basically we have dualistic vision; that is ignorance and through that ignorance we always believe that objects and an "I" or a subject exist. Through dualistic vision we have this body. Our body also came about through ignorance. If we did not have this ignorance since the beginning we would not have this physical body and also we would not have to suffer in samsara. So, ignorance is the fundamental basis of our existence.

What do we need to do? We need to put all our energy and all our efforts into recognizing or discovering our ignorance. It is guaranteed that if we find our ignorance we can certainly find the antidote for it. Ignorance does have an antidote; that's for sure. What is the best we can do now as humans? We have a very smart, sharp mind, plus we have the teaching and there are still teachers in the world; so we should use this opportunity to pursue the teaching, to discover our ignorance and to find the antidote to it.

As we said before, the cause of emotional and mental disease is an imbalance of the *lung* or wind element. So now we need to know the particular conditions that directly activate *lung* disorders. As we said yesterday and the day before, in general there are four types of conditions: diet, behavior, seasonal changes, and provocations.

In general when we look at our samsara, on our planet nowadays there are a lot of improvements in our lives, but there are also a lot of wars and poverty. Even though Europe and America are developed countries many people are seeking enjoyment and happiness by using drugs, drinking alcohol, or sometimes changing religion and so forth. These kinds of changes bring a lot of side effects. And when we look at what we consider Third World or underdeveloped countries or still developing countries like India, we see they also have a lot of problems. One is the problem of how to survive. Then there is a lot of theft, murder, robbery, and violence. People even have to worry about the police: the police are supposed to protect their lives, but they also sometimes become like mafia. In India there is a joke: they say the police are authorized robbers; they have like a license for robbery.

Through this kind of life, always living with fear, people get exhausted, or stressed and, gradually accumulating this, they get sick. In some places, just to survive, to keep alive, you have to do certain things you don't like, for example killing animals. You do not like doing it, but you have to do it for survival or to support your family. Also sometimes you have to do certain things verbally that you do not like, such as lying. So also this kind of thing causes disease. It doesn't matter whether you live in a developed country or an underdeveloped one, everybody is equally seeking happiness.

Also we all think that happiness is something we can get from outside, like an object, and that as soon as we find it we'll get happiness. People have this kind of attitude. That's why they are always looking for happiness outside. If we think that happiness comes from an object, even if we get that object we are never satisfied; we need more and more, and so our pursuit of the objects for giving us happiness never ends.

I'll tell you a story. It is a very ancient story, but it is relevant. There was a teacher and a student. They had some gold. They were carrying it on a journey to the center of Tibet. The teacher was always telling the student: "Do not sleep, try not to sleep!" and also he was trying to stay awake himself. So they had a very difficult journey trying to protect the gold. One day the student told the teacher: "Tonight we can sleep peacefully." So the teacher thought that maybe he had found another person to protect the gold and asked the student, "Why?" The student replied, "I threw away the gold". [laughter] This is a story, but if we apply it in our life it makes a lot of sense. Whatever we have, whether we have power, wealth, or fame, we are never satisfied, and that gives tremendous suffering. For example, if we have an itch we think that if we scratch it we'll feel better, but if you scratch it you'll need to scratch more. The more you scratch the more it itches. In the same way any kind of desire is never satisfied.

Through this kind of ignorance if you see someone better off than yourself, you become jealous; if someone is worse off than you, you feel proud. If someone is equal, on the same level, then you ignore him. So through this kind of mistaken attitude we can get all kinds of problems. If we look really closely this is scientific. For example, if you are attracted to someone and you cannot get that person then you have jealousy or anger toward the person who can get what you want. Then you sort of blame that person and this often leads to violence. So, when we see things as objects, those objects make us distracted; and through distraction we have attachment.

Where does attachment come from? The brain is the organ or factor that creates attachment. As soon as we see an object our brain either accepts or rejects it; either way these are big emotional and mental and energy movements. Scientists know that very well, so I am not going to talk about it today. When the brain engages in excessive attachment or rejection, it creates something like movement or circulation. This movement creates patterns that lead to the accumulation of something like a residue. So in the brain we've accumulated the residue of every emotion. This residue later leaks down, like water dripping, and those drops could go into the heart, into the lungs and into every organ. In scientific labs today we can see the measurements of the amounts of stress in the blood. So I feel that today's science laboratory work is very good for introducing and explaining ancient knowledge, making a sort of understandable language to introduce it to people.

In Tibetan medicine we say that *peken*, which is translated as phlegm, is located in the upper part of the body, in the brain. *Peken* has the nature of the earth and water elements. Even though it is located in the upper part of the body the function drips down into the whole body. We say that, but we do not have anything like scientific proof of how it drips or where it drips; we know it through the symptoms. Today in the lab we can actually *see* how many cells there are in the blood, how many cells in the muscles and so on, so then we can tell that it is true what the ancient Tibetan medicine says, that the earth and water elements drip down into the body. I do not know so much about science, but I really like it.

Now what happens is that emotions make a sort of impure residue and the accumulation of this impure residue makes the body sick. The result of bodily sickness or the result of a bodily dysfunction feeds back to the emotions and the emotions make unhappiness, anxiety, and so forth. So these two make something like an alliance with each other; they have an interdependent relationship. When we look at mind or consciousness and body they are two different things. But consciousness is located in the body, so as long as these two support each other they are functioning. But sometimes one of them has a dysfunction and the other is affected by it; this makes a type of sickness called psychosomatic or mental illness.

When we compare bodily suffering with mental suffering, we find that mental suffering is much worse than bodily suffering. Sometimes we can observe a person who seems very poor, in poor health and with a very poor style of living, but we can see how that person is living his life, singing, dancing, and looking very happy. So how does the physical aspect affect mental health? If you have physical problems how do they affect the emotions? I will tell you a very short story. Sorry, I am a storyteller [laughter]. The story comes from India. I like stories, but I'll try to make it short.

A very poor mother and her son were living on the lower end of a street and a king was living up the hill. Ancient Indian kings used to ride on an elephant when they went on outings. So the mother and son were living on the street where the king used to pass. The man in charge of the king's elephant used to take it up and down that street every day. He never succeeded in bringing the elephant to the king on time; he was late every day. One day the king asked why, what was the cause. He answered that on the street he had to pass two beggars, a mother and her son, and the little boy would always hold onto the tail of the elephant so it couldn't move. That was his reason, his excuse for arriving late [laughter].

The king thought it was a little strange. He did not punish the elephant minder but sent his ministers to check who that boy was. They found the son. He was a skinny little thing. The ministers asked the boy: "Where is your house? Take us to your mother!" and he did. When they arrived they saw the house was just a grass roof. The minister asked the mother about her life and what she was feeding the boy. The mother answered that sometimes she could find a little bread and sometimes she could not find even that. The minister reported that information to the king. Then the king sent someone to bring the mother to the palace and he said to her, "Now bring me what you give your son to eat." She made the bread that she was normally giving to her son and eating herself and gave it to the king. The king could not eat it, it was uneatable. The king asked how her son was so strong that when he held the tail of the elephant it could not move and what was the reason for that. The mother answered: "In general, whether or not we have food, I tell my son not to worry. And also I don't tell him if tomorrow we will not have any food." So the king realized how important the mind is to the body and told the mother that, starting from the next day, in case of no food, she should tell her son, "Tomorrow we will not have any food." So, starting from the third day, the elephant arrived to the king precisely on time. Once the boy found that the next day there would not be any food he started to worry thinking: "I might be hungry tomorrow, and my mother too." This kind of worry made his body weak; so when he was trying to hold the tail of the elephant he didn't have any strength, and the elephant arrived on time.

What this story is telling us is that worrying is useless because even if we worry the conditions don't change. Also Shantideva said: "If something can be fixed then you don't need to worry about it. If there is no way to fix things it is useless to worry, worrying doesn't help." This is really true. If we apply that information to daily life it will be of great benefit to our health.

In Tibetan medicine we say that every individual has a kind of vital essence that we call *dang*. The *dang* is very important for maintaining our life, to keep our body and mind peaceful and functioning. But there are different causes of losing the *dang*. One of the main causes is the mind. If you have stress, unhappiness, sadness, suffering, that is the main cause for losing the *dang*. The short story I told you is like a proof of what is said in Tibetan medicine: that *dang* is important for health and that worrying is the cause for losing it.

Worry is fundamental to bringing suffering to individuals, families, communities, society; it is the root of all suffering. The root of worry is attachment. For that reason Buddha said it is a poison. Whatever name we give an illness, Alzheimer's, depression, anxiety, or whatever, the root is basically the same: unhappiness. The cause is one, but there are various symptoms of the body and also different levels of symptoms. If we could understand that attachment is the root of all these diseases and problems that would bring great benefit.

I am not saying that attachment is not good in the sense that we should be monks and go live in the mountains to practice; that is not a solution. It is also not important whether or not you believe there are future lives. What is important is that we see today, in a practical way, that attachment brings a lot of suffering. To avoid attachment completely is not so easy, but if you know that it brings suffering, that it brings unwanted results, that is already a big help.

Now I will tell you another story. During the time of the 7th Dalai Lama, a wealthy, powerful man from China asked a Tibetan man, "Who in Tibet is the symbol of a homeless practitioner who avoids attachment to all material things?" The man answered: "The 7th Dalai Lama, His Holiness Kalsang Gyatso." The Chinese man had a big shock because the 7th Dalai Lama was living in the Potala Palace, surrounded by ministers and assistants. He thought, how does he come to be unattached to material things? Maybe you people are shocked too. If we really think well, we can understand that it is the truth. It is similar to the lotus flower that grows in muddy water, but the flower is never muddy; it is very pure, clean. Similarly, we need to live in samsara, in our circumstances; but if we know the result or effect of attachment, even if we live in samsara, we remain pure. If you know this, firstly it makes you peaceful; secondly your peaceful mind makes you happy and healthy. If your mind is peaceful and happy, your body is healthy, and you will be able to build a healthy, happy family. A healthy, happy family can build a happy, healthy society or community. So what do you think? Is that something good? Then we should move in that direction.

Now we make it more simple. We do have methods of diagnosis in Tibetan medicine in the clinical aspect of mental diseases. As Doctor Phuntsog mentioned yesterday we have many methods also for diagnosis. For example, firstly we search for the cause of the disease; secondly we observe the symptoms; and thirdly we observe the effects or benefits of the therapies. There are many ways we can observe or diagnose.

This morning the presenters also explained the importance of the environment, the family, and the lifestyle. These also are part of the diagnosis, where the disease is coming from, so I am not going to repeat that. Observation of the symptoms can include many things. We observe all the symptoms through the person's reactions and also by using the equipment or instruments for diagnosis. So, we diagnose by using many different kinds of methods, and equipment as well as by observing the symptoms.

The next and most important part is prevention. Today everybody agrees that prevention is more important than treatment. For example, there are many programs on diet and nutrition. I think all of them are very good. I totally agree with them.

Another aspect we explained before is the cause and condition the disease. When something happens to us we always blame other people; we always act as if we are innocent and blame others. We do not have the power, it is not easy to change that idea because we have the *habit* of always blaming others when something bad happens. But if we have the capacity or the opportunity it is good to try to learn how to change this attitude; not to always say someone else is bad, but to look inside ourselves. For example, if you are about to get a good salary and someone says something to your boss and you get less than what you were supposed to get, if somehow they caused you not accomplish your goal, for sure you will get angry. But if you think well, before he tried to harm you, maybe you started to harm him, so now he is sort of repaying. If you look well, yes, the problem is from him this time, but in origin *I* made some problems for him so he is now repaying or getting revenge. The cause, the root is me. It is important to try not to harm any human being, any sentient being. There is also a practice of the Lojong or training of the mind. This kind of practice is very important to prevent the disease.

As I said before we should not put the blame on other people. Why? Because all our modern facilities, all this fancy life we enjoy nowadays comes from the global population, all sentient beings have worked for it in their own different ways: wealthy people with money, smart people with knowledge, and so on. With all that put together today we have this peaceful, harmonious society with many facilities, in this life. When we think about this we should thank everybody, even though I am working, even though I am doing business, even though I have to make a living. Of course, if someone's life depends on someone else he should thank that person, that is normal. But we should thank all sentient beings in the world as well.

A professor might be said to be a great scholar, but if he or she does not have any students, where does this fame come from? A famous professor needs students, they are important because they give him that opportunity. So if we use this as a kind of model, whenever we have some problems we'll always think: "Oh, that's good"; whenever something good happens to us we'll think: "Oh, that is good." If we have this kind of attitude, even if we have some suffering, the suffering will be a little lighter, less heavy. With this kind of attitude we can have a method to prevent disease and we can have a healthy body.

Some people accept the whole philosophy of rebirth, and they follow a path to become enlightened so as to be able to help to free all sentient beings from suffering. But if there are no other sentient beings, for whom are you going to practice that help? You cannot become enlightened without sentient beings. Where does the enlightenment come from? That is also an interdependent relationship. That is also part of the treatment.

Now I am going to stop here, thank you all for listening.

(4th session)

Dr. Francisco Barnosell Pi earned a degree in medicine and surgery in 1976 and received his doctor from the School of Medicine of the University of Barcelona in 1981. He specialized in rehabilitation, neurology, and electromyography. He has been head of service in medical units specializing in neurological diagnosis tests at various clinics and hospitals in Catalonia.

He is currently research director of the Integrative Medicine Association and author of the book *Entre dos aguas: Experiencias de un médico sobre las terapias alternativas* [Sitting on the Fence: experiences of a doctor with alternative therapies] published by Editorial Luciérnaga (Planeta, 2012). He is also a member of various NGOs and associations, where he researches the effects of ancestral medicines. He has brought together physicians, healers, and therapists in a pioneering conference held in Barcelona in 2013.

PRESENTATION

FRANCISCO BARNOSELL
Differential Diagnosis in Dementia
or Schizophrenia by Applying an Integrative
Approach: A Personal View

I would like to thank the organizers; thank you, Carmen; special thanks to the Tibetan School of Medicine and to the Fundació Uszheimer for having succeeded in creating this great family, for allowing us to talk about topics that are not easy. Yesterday I was very pleased when during the roundtable we diverged from the subject to talk about the legal aspect. It is a genuine cause of concern that as conventional physicians we are "playing around" with therapies that are not fully recognized by the official schools. This has always been a problem, but I believe we need to have the courage to do so with a lot of respect so that we can be listened to. And of course I agree with Sergio Abanades that it is very important to do it from *within* the system because if we don't, we will not change anything. Since I've noticed that we like stories, and that is the easiest way to make people understand, this is my story:

I am a conventional physician; I still work in mainstream medicine. I am a neurophysiologist, neurologist, and rehabilitation physician, and I apply a diagnosis technique called electromyography, a neuromuscular technique or test used to assess the health of the peripheral nervous system. In other words, I continue to work in this field, but for more than ten years now I have been investigating alternative, complementary therapies, now called integrative therapies (I love how the name keeps changing). Our point of view and our life circumstances change us; in other words, all of us here will not be the same tomorrow. Why? Because of our interactions with one another, and the changes these inputs bring about.

This is a picture of me with the machine I work with in one of the clinics and the people who have changed my perspective as a physician. Milagros Herrera is a channeler, and here below – with this hairstyle that I wear in summer – I am standing next to Alex Orbito, Jean Jacques Breluzeau, and Olivier. They are healers, medicine men, mediums. They have perceptions that others don't have. I need to use these first five minutes of the presentation to explain a little about myself to those who don't know me, since later I will get into the topic of differential diagnosis of dementias, schizophrenias, from the point of view of integrative medicine. Most cases are erroneously diagnosed, but in order for you to believe me, I must explain my experiences a little so you can understand why I have wound up here. It will take only five minutes.

When I was in Asia, I served as a guinea pig for a healer who is able to insert his hands inside the body, the open body, without anesthesia, without anything, and who has the capacity to materialize a situation, or the energetic part of the illness, which he then takes away.

I am going to show you a very short video just so you see how the perspective of a Western physician, with classic studies, changes and will never be the same after watching situations like these. This is but a small example. Here I am with Jean Jacques; I made him come. He lives on Île de Ré but travels around the world. He is a geobiologist who uses the Lecher antenna as a diagnosis tool. The Lecher antenna looks like the Egyptian ankh cross, and so with a movement of his hands he is able to calibrate the Bovis energy of a situation, of a question he asks. I have had patients with illnesses that couldn't be diagnosed and who were sent away from several care services. I told him: "I am going to take two or three of these patients to see if we can get a diagnosis."

Jean Jacques is not a physician. So here we have the example of this man, and thanks to him we did the correct diagnosis of a pathology that could not be labeled medically.

Why am I saying this? Because I have learned a lot from therapists, from healers; they are people who are many years ahead of us, and conventional medicine has not given them the respect they deserve. I have been investigating them for over ten years now and every time I am more surprised. How did all this start? With my blog on medicine and therapies. I started it under the name Paco La Cueva because I felt like I was hiding in a cave; I was a little afraid to get out in the open. But ladies and gentlemen, in the three years that this blog has been around, there have been more than 300,000 entries.

When this happens you realize there is a strong interest in people to find out about other types of medicine. The day I appeared in the newspaper stating that healers and physicians should collaborate with each other, 21,000 entries were posted on my blog, and I received thousands of emails, more than 2,000 in a single day. Now I receive around 300 emails every week. Imagine having to manage these emails coming from all over the world from patients, healers, therapists, regular people, physicians, and extraordinary physicians who are working in hospitals in a conventional way but who have different perceptions that they do not dare talk about for fear of being ostracized. All this resulted in interviews such as this one on the left, about a physician who is trying to build that bridge between the different medical approaches. It also inspired my book *Entre dos aguas* where, like a reporter, I explain many events. Finally, I created the Asociación de Médicos y Sanadores (Association of Physicians and Healers). I expressly did not include the word "therapists" in this name. Instead I used "healers" because I wanted to move more toward the liberal side, toward people who really do unimaginable things, who work in that invisible form of medicine that cannot be demonstrated, where there is no magnetic resonance imaging, no ultrasound scanning, no analysis to prove it, but that provides results in the end. Those results translate into improved health for the patient, sometimes spectacular improvement.

These people have changed my life. I met these six people and within a short time, I organized a conference and got to know them better. To think that this conference was organized in a few days; there was an audience of almost 700 people. Can you imagine this? Seven hundred people interested in this combined medicine, and around 30% of them were physicians.

Of course, I received many calls from all kinds of people asking me how I managed to bring together in one location, in one room, physicians who are willing to talk to therapists and healers. It was by simply answering those thousands of emails sent by brave people who wished to be there. Curiously, the person who moderated that event, Dr. Martínez, is here too. My perception of each person here has changed me; has changed my circumstances and what I think. I believe that it is very important to unite science and the heart, the soul, the spirit. We are more than just one body; this has been mentioned quite a few times in this forum, and spirituality, morality and lifestyles are essential since that, ultimately, is what is changing us, the way we see things. Now I would like to show you a video.

I am the patient, I was suffering from phlebitis. You can see the healer, he breaks the skin with the hands, and is able to materialize the area with the clot; he doesn't take out the damaged area, we can say he removes it through the skin, materializing it. I am not going to go on with this topic because it would be a little complicated.

I have another video. I am showing it here so you can see how a conventional physician, with his machines, his university, his courses, his conferences, suddenly goes to Asia to take a course, forgets that he is a physician, takes off his white coat and sees a case – it could be a cancer, an aneurism, a tumor, a psychological problem, Alzheimer's, all sorts of problems – then suddenly he sees that the healer has cured that person, and that many other, not all, got better. Of course I say to myself "How is this possible? This has not been taught at my college! What am I doing here!" And I am standing there with a silly look on my face, telling myself "all my science… all my papers, presentations… all my publications… It's not possible, I don't believe it." I have the greatest respect for anyone who is able to heal in this way. Later, I theorized about this. I have seen hundreds, over one thousand operations of this kind, also performed by other healers who have taught me that there is another medicine. It is important to mention that.

This is me [again]; I suffered from a herniated cervical disk, which was very painful, and as a result of this operation the truth is that the pain was gone. The injury was caused by a serious motorcycle accident; I was in a coma. Time went by and when I was in the Philippines I took advantage of the occasion and told the healer "Try to cure me of this." But then I also suffered from a herniated lumbar disk, you will see now, watch what he is removing, the material he is removing, because I will compare it with a surgery I had later that was performed by the traumatologist. It is the same texture. It is pink, isn't it? Well, if someone is capable of doing this, and other things, how could you not believe what I will explain to you now about dementias and so on. I had three hernias; the healer removed one of them the pain came back and I ended up with the traumatologist when I returned. This is what he removed, which is pretty much the same as that removed by the healer. There's no need for words, this is an image. I placed myself in this situation in order to experience it and then be able to explain it.

What all this mounts up to is that orthodox medicine is not at odds with the research of other new paradigms. An open, scrupulous mind is required. Now I will start to talk about my perceptions regarding dementias or schizophrenias, which in the examples I will show you were incorrectly diagnosed as such. It could be that it takes a shift in perception to understand the experiences I will now explain that involve highly sophisticated situations – at shamanic and healing levels. Following less rigid guidelines in the diagnoses, we enter this world of emotions, of perceptions. A different sensitivity is required to diagnose other possibilities with patience. One needs to be courageous, be a good listener above all, and have what here in Catalonia we call *sentit comú*, or common sense, since this is really very helpful. But it seems it has been lost lately because we live in a mad world that doesn't give us time, not even to have normal relationships with each other. When you need to find anything on the Internet and you enter a word, you get like 100,000 results, so how are you going to look at even ten of them.

I am going to talk about cases of diagnostic errors of dementias or schizophrenias, including the full names of the patients. Thanks to the fact that I have been involved in this world of alternative medicine, now called integrative medicine, I have been able to delve into the subject, especially with people I have met on the way and who have explained it to me, in particular through those blogs you have seen, which were mostly written by physicians and healers, and through the emails from regular people, even people of an advanced age, who had never before revealed to anybody what they were able to see, to perceive. These are people with different perceptions and sensitivities; they hear sounds, voices, music, see visual effects with lights, colors. I believe they have a special gift. We all have some special gift, but they surpass us; their special gifts go beyond those of the majority of people. Their psychology is usually a little distorted because these are people who have suffered greatly in order to be understood by their surroundings. So in the end, as a physician, you say, "Well, they have access to a dimension and we lack the key that would allow us to enter there."

Therefore, the problem is that medicine – conventional medicine – misdiagnoses them and treats them as if they had psychological pathologies. They endure terrible internal struggles to move forward, meet with a total lack of understanding from those around them, and find refuge in religion, art, writing, philosophy, especially as a means, a safety valve. But they are great in those areas.

However, these are people who are afraid of looking within themselves and finding that double face, so others don't discover that they are different. It is as easy as saying: "Well, ladies and gentlemen, I have this special gift, don't worry." At the conference organized by the Association [of Physicians and Healers] here in Barcelona, last September, I was glad to see that for the first time at least there were people who during their presentation publicly stated: "Yes, I have this special gift and now I am able to say so." It could be premonition, seeing lights, seeing beings, any type of special gift, but the important point is to acknowledge it, to say it publicly, and that the person sitting right next to him or her does not say: "You're mad." That is very important for them and for the type of society we have to live in, one that appreciates minorities and is respectful of those who are different.

OK, here you can see some people, including their full names. I asked for their permission first so I could talk about them publicly. I spoke to them and they were very pleased, because these are people who have suffered a great deal. I am not going to explain each case because there's no time. These are people who have been in psychiatric hospitals. More than one person underwent psychological tests for years and in the end more than 80% of those who appear here were labeled as schizophrenic, paranoid, ill, and yet they are people who are absolutely normal – I have met all of them – but with different perceptions.

I wanted to call the attention of this forum to the fact that we must be careful when we make diagnoses because there are people who are different, but that doesn't mean that we have to label them as having pathologies, which is really very serious considering what they have experienced. Like Rosa March, who, ever since she was a child, was able to see lights, see auras, and have perceptions that were impossible to explain; or like Rosa Gaite, who had the advantage of at least being understood by her family, who said, "Well, don't say it outside the home because it won't look good." She was a girl, who, for example, said one evening, "Tonight Aunt Maria will come." "But she is in Madrid and we are in living in the Basque Country, quite far away." "She will come tonight." And the aunt arrived. She had that perception; she was able to access that world, that dimension, through a connection we don't know about.

The one you see above, Rosa March, was really punished and much vilified by the doctors through their diagnoses just because she would say that she saw things that others don't see.

Milagros Herrera beats them all since she is someone who channels; to channel means that the person enters another dimension, where she obtains information that others can't access. When Milagros was eight, she grabbed her father's leg and cried "Don't leave, don't leave." The father thought she was upset and was throwing a tantrum; she kept grabbing her father's leg for a certain period of time, until she finally let go of it. The father hit her. Well, because of the many things she perceived and saw, she was locked up in a mental institution for more than six months. She went through all the doctors, psychiatrists, and psychologists and took every test possible, but nothing was found. After grabbing her father's leg and begging him not to leave, the family learned that the bus the father would have taken had fallen off a cliff and everyone inside was killed. She saw that something like that would happen to her father if he rode that bus. Of course, this had to happen in order for it to be credible.

I have experienced hundreds of cases like these. I have included only eight here, but I have done it for all of you who are involved in the world of dementias, Alzheimer's, schizophrenia, to encourage you to think that there are people who are different and that that doesn't mean we have to label them. Like Mimón Sancho, who said she able to speak with plants. Of course, when I met her, I was very young and was not yet a physician; I thought "She is nuts. I speak with plants? Sure!" I've come to know her better over the years; she is a floral therapist now. Somehow she gets the information about the plants her patient requires; but there is no need to go looking in Tibet, China, or South America for plants that grow in those places only. She walks around the city and picks two flowers from a pot located in a specific place, and these flowers have the precise resonance to cure the illness of a patient who came to see her that same afternoon. That is the advantage of the place and location, like going to do the shopping next door.

Lluis Coll [was considered] a strange boy. He was placed in a boarding school for eight years because at a young age he used to cure other children by placing his hands on them when they hurt themselves. The family was very frightened, so he spent time in that school for being a "strange" boy. Can you imagine the eight-year ordeal he had to go through simply because he was a perceptive person? Now he is a great shaman. Let me tell you what he told me yesterday, just a detail, an example, since he has explained many things to me, I've had the honor of working with him. Keep in mind that Lluis cleans trains for a living; he is a simple person but his capacity as a healer is enormous and nobody can see what he sees. A friend we have in common called him yesterday and said, "Hey, Lluis, I fell down and hurt myself on my side. I went to the hospital but they didn't find anything wrong." All this was going on over the phone. Lluis said, "Hold on a minute," then he put his hand on his own side and said, "Oh, tell them to take a look at the fifth rib on the right side, because I think there is a fissure." Our friend said, "No, no, they have already looked, and nothing is wrong." He then called me. "Paco, Lluis told me" and so on. "Lluis said that? Go get an X-ray." He had the X-ray done again and I recommended other tests as well. The fissure was found – over the phone. When I see things like this I say to myself, "What is a magnetic resonance imaging for?"

I am giving you two examples but I have been experiencing strange cases like these every day for more than ten years now. So, of course, the fact that I am still working as a physician, is amazing, right?

Maite Díaz was quite a normal girl; she discovered a little late in life that she resonates with her voice. With her voice she is able to vibrate the pathology resonance of the patient, and she cures patients with mantras. Then there is Rosamari Ramirez. All these people spoke at the conference. It is really remarkable to see children who are mediums in a conference of physicians and healers. How do we recognize them? Because she is a medium, she is able to recognize them. Of course, it's a great [gift], because when a mother would come to see me with her child, a strange boy, I could not be sure about the child, but she could because she was one of them and has experienced, well, very drastic situations. Rosamari discovered it late in life; she was thirty-some years old. As a result of an illness, something incredible happened. It's as if her mind had removed a curtain and suddenly she started to have all kind of perceptions, visualizations, and premonitions, but of an excellent quality. The day I met her, not long ago, she told me several things over the phone that would happen. I was really astonished. Not even two months passed when everything she told me came true… I thought, well, I better not ask any more since all this is very dangerous.

Laia Rovira underwent all kinds of medical tests, absolutely all of them. She was really in a very complicated family environment because nobody believed her and she was considered mad, paranoid, in a delusional state, because of the things she could see. Luckily, she had a brother who started having the same experiences when he grew up, so the family thought "Gosh! If he is like her, let's not be so harsh." And that was the great advantage; sad, though, having to wait until you are more than 30 years old before others believe you.

What has happened? Many physicians and nurses have contacted me; the last communication was, I think, a couple of days ago, at the clinic where I work. One of the nurses was scared; she told me that when she is working in the intensive care unit she sees not only the patient but also beings surrounding the patient. "Paco, what should I do?" And I replied: "What do you want me to say? You are in a clinic so keep on working!" [Laughter in audience.] Yes, we may laugh at these situations, but for the person who is working there and is experiencing it directly, it is really hard. At the beginning I was very worried because I thought "Goodness! Of course, things like these must happen in clinics all the time." But imagine those people with special gifts or who have those perceptions, if they reveal them openly, they are labeled in an inappropriate way, to say the least. Many children talk about an imaginary friend. We have all heard this from small children. When they grow up this friend goes away, but some remain. Another striking example is the case of twins. What happens with twins? One is home with the mother and the other goes out. The mother says "Dear me, it's two in the morning and he is not here. Maybe he's been in a motorcycle accident?" And the twin says "No, mother, don't worry, he's all right." So he can perceive that his twin brother is all right. What kind of connection makes him say that his twin is fine when they are kilometers apart? And when one twin is ill, the other wakes up with a start and tells her mother "He is not well, something is wrong." We are talking about situations that medicine is unable to explain logically. We should investigate these situations since surely one thing will lead us to another.

There are elderly people, 85 years old, who have written in my blog for the first time in their lives – they belong to well-known families in Barcelona – and they are the kind of people we have been talking about, but they had never said it before; they even have great-grandchildren, and if they would reveal it now their families would say they have Alzheimer's. But the only thing they have is the perceptions they had during their whole life but did not dare reveal.

Where is all this taking us? To reflect on the real origin of medicine, of illness. We have an overly rigid vision; we have to be more flexible and not react with stress since it stimulates and disturbs the system. I loved what Lobsang said about those stories he told. I can add one more, about morals, the morals we all have. To go against the inner commitments we make as human beings is what often causes an illness. I will give a simple example. Someone is a person of integrity when it comes to family matters but maybe at work, due to his specialty he has to lie, or act incorrectly; that kind of duality will damage his body because his cells know that 70% of the time he is acting correctly but 30% of the time he is lying or altering things because maybe it is good for business, such as a car salesman, when he says the vehicle is fantastic and the engine is totally damaged. He knows he is lying but his cells know it too, and that duality creates internal systems that may be the start of an illness. It is an iceberg, and iceberg that cannot be seen. OK, I'm going to go through these slides quickly. I have the advantage of being the last speaker and many things have already been said. As for what is written on this slide, *combination of therapies*, that topic is obsolete at this point, right?

A global vision of the patient: This is really important; to show patients how to manage their situation, being conscious of *their* reality. The reality of the patient, not the way that we, as specialists, believe it should be. We have to put ourselves in their shoes and see with their eyes, only then will we understand what lies behind the illness.

Body, mind, emotions, and spirit: Not long ago this was a big novelty; today anyone who doesn't believe it is like someone who isn't able to speak English.

Lifestyle and living environment: How each person lives is very important and this is connected with the morals I just referred to. Another factor is the direct environment and the amount of electromagnetic pollution that surrounds us, such as WiFi, radios, phones, those remote-control red lights that follow you around the house. All this affects our health.

This is why I was interested in attending this fantastic forum, a family that was formed here swiftly since there was little time to organize it, and I was interested to talk about some of the diagnosed cases like the ones I have shown you including the patients' full names. There are many more that I have not been able to present because time is limited, and these people have written many emails telling me about the hard times they endured only because they are sensitive and perceptive and have special gifts that the rest of us don't have and see the world differently.

Responsibility: It must be reciprocal and shared. We must involve the patient completely; if not, we will fail to achieve that connection, which is necessary for improving health. In particular, we need to empower the innate capacity of the body to recover by itself. I am convinced that there is a spot we haven't discovered yet, and that when you touch that like when resetting a phone the default codes are restored again. We need to find that spot because we could then restore the codes we had when we were born and recuperate that indispensable information again. And as Lobsang was saying before, we also have those residues that remain inside of us. It would be fantastic to be able to find that reset spot and the way to go back to our original condition.

Ladies and gentleman, as for *an open mind for evolution*, anything can be said if it is said with respect and, of course, given our age, since most of us are getting older, I believe we can say everything we need to say respectfully in any forum. We are physicians; we are working, researching, and we accept new paradigms. Why not? What matters is not just experience and research but also that patients are really healed and cured.

The healing effect: I am not going to talk about this now since I've done that already, but I will mention the need to change the quality of the patient's healing ritual. Today, physicians rarely touch their patients, they don't touch them! Moreover, our system, lately, when you leave the doctor's office is to say, "OK, you can leave now, the consultation is over." The doctor has barely looked at the patient or touched him. You go to another area, where a machine is waiting, and then the machine gives you the prescription. The prescription! The sacred act of the doctor-patient union! The doctor says, "Take this medicine" so that the patient will believe that it works. Now you head to a machine and push a button, and in four days time – for a certain amount of euros because if you don't pay, the prescription won't come out – the prescription will be ready and will tell you what you need to do. I believe that from the psychological point of view we are breaking a lot of chains in order for the system to work. Well, that's just the way it is. There is a crisis; we need to maybe reduce the number of bureaucrats in some places. We need more physicians, but they give us more politicians. And we have to think of the consequences for our health, not only ours but also for future generations. I am not talking about genetics.

OK, I think we really must mention two people who at least in my opinion are important in connection with what I have learned and found. They are David Rakel, in the United States, one of the pioneers of integrative medicine, and Juan Carlos Duran, an oncologist who works in the Canary Islands, a fighter with incredible energy. He is already setting up integrative medicine there, and is speaking loud and clear about what many do not dare say. I have deepest respect for both of them.

What has happened in time? Eventually, I established this association of physicians and healers, and I managed to get physicians to come and speak at this conference. And let's not forget something that I think is essential, that therapists are years ahead of us; they have investigated, have attended courses, have done things that physicians discover only later. That's why I have included them on the same level as physicians, so no one is more important than the other and they can all have the opportunity to speak at the conference about various topics like the ones we have heard as well as other subjects I am reluctant to discuss here for fear of being ostracized. Examples include how to send lost souls toward the light. In my case, as a physician, I am very interested in the destiny of the soul. I am a physician but destiny is vital because in the formula, in the equation of illness, to include the word "destiny" may change my perspective completely on how to situate myself in relation to this patient. I will fight for the patient's life until the last second but the perception of the illness changes if I include destiny in the equation.

We have formed 30 research teams. It's a mixed bag because the important thing was not to direct people to this or that pathology. "What do you do most?" "I see cases of autism." "OK, put together an autism team; find a physician, a healer, a therapist, and form the team." Then a lot of people would sign up. "And you, who do you see?" "I see cases of arthritis." "OK, an arthritis team." The interesting thing is that this is about teams that carry out research activities the same way as in a clinic or hospital, based on medical morale and ethics, but incorporating therapists and healers in these activities since they work differently. For example, in cancer cases, Reiki, biomagnetism, polarity, metamorphic techniques, or Ho'oponopono may be applied. Of course, we physicians don't know about this but therapists do know. This is why it is very important to unite physicians and therapists so we may learn from each other. These teams are increasing day by day since I receive emails daily. We started a week ago and there are thirty of us already, and I still have many to post. I think that by the end of the month we will be around one hundred.

We are continuing with integrative medicine courses and we will hold our second conference in the last week of June.

Finally, I have two gifts for the audience. This is the first gift: There is a country that includes legal provisions on integrative medicine in legislature. As we already know, the World Health Organization now recognizes integrative medicine. However, which country comes forward and states that it can be applied and practiced together with conventional medicine? Except for one country, for legal and official reasons, hardly any other acknowledges integrative medicine. I was surprised to see in an article that this country's laws consider human beings to be "a unity of the universe." This is a very advanced concept, politically speaking. It also mentions energetic illnesses. This country is Nicaragua.

Harmonic relationship of balance and awareness that we are one; we are energy: When I said in an interview that "we are energy moved by chemistry," meaning chemistry and electrical impulses, you have no idea how many emails I received from physicists and chemists asking me if I was crazy. Well, it can't be proven, but there it is. And then it turns out that [Nicaragua] dared to enact a law about it; and most importantly, shamanic medicine is also considered. We have so much to learn from ancestral medicine, which dates back thousands of years. These are things we did not learn about in college, but rather later on. I believe that now we have opened this Pandora's box it won't be closed ever again, and it will lead us to unexpected places.

Let me show you some images of an experience with an energetic pyramid, when I gathered 17 channelers together; each one, individually, had to explain to me, using paper and pencil, what they saw when I was carrying out a healing process inside the circle. You would be astounded at the thing these persons are able to see; visual effects when you are placing your hands on the patient without even touching him; the things they can see even inside organs. That is why, based on experiences such as these that I have had, I dare say with regard to the topic I introduced today that many diagnostic errors have been made. Be careful with people with different sensitivities! The body is more than just a body; it is mind, spirituality, fields, emotions, perceptions, and all this moves as vibrations. These bodies are like different dresses we wear one on top of the other. We need to believe it, with faith, even though there is no magnetic resonance imaging, no analysis telling us this exists. But it is essential to acknowledge these things. Here is my book; I will be glad to talk about it later.

Finally, *the medicine of the future* will talk about vibrations, sunlight, photonic energy.

Above all, most importantly, the last thing, *to believe is to create*. If we can manage not to materialize our thoughts according to each situation, we will keep illnesses away.

I am a physician. My name is Francisco Barnosell. I am a neurologist, neurophysiologist, a rehabilitation physician and – I say this with much pride – I am doing research into astral surgery. Thank you very much.

(5th session)

ROUNDTABLE

Ms. Neus Rodríguez, Dr. Guillem Martí, Dr. Lobsang Tenzin,
Dr. Francisco Barnosell

Moderator: Dr. Carmen Martinez

Moderator: We are reaching the end of this extraordinary conference where we have shared our knowledge. For me it was an astonishing experience to discover that we were talking about virtually the same things, but with different words. Yesterday I was amazed by the talk about the three poisons, especially the poison of ignorance. I think, and I really feel, after forty years of practicing medicine, that ignorance of who we are, what we are doing here, and what is the purpose of our existence – ignorance of our spiritual purpose in this life – is ultimately what is causing our diseases.

So, let's open the discussion about these very interesting talks. If you have a comment or question, go ahead.

Rodriguez: I want to make my contribution. We have talked about patients and about caregivers, but we should also be talking about those who take care of the caregivers. We should always try to guarantee help or support for them. As Guillem Martí explained this morning, those who are caring for dependent patients forget to take care of themselves because they are caring for someone else. So, of course we have to stress the need of help for them and sometimes they need guidance. That is what we do in our foundation: we provide guidance so that caregivers do not end up ill or sick themselves. We have to care for them, because they are also suffering emotionally. For example, can you imagine how a daughter feels when she has to start commanding her father? She has to change her role. This is so hard because her father was her support, and now she has to support him. Of course, the caregivers need a lot of the therapies and different medicines that were talked about in this conference. I think that we should stress this more, because sometimes only the patients and the caregivers are aware of the problems they are suffering, but not the people around them.

Twenty years ago only the family members of the patients would come to us, but now that we have more information the patients themselves come to us seeking help. That is an improvement. Of course we give support to people around them. These are things that have changed.

One thing that did not change is the ignorance. People still do not know what to do in these situations: how they can manage their emotions, their suffering. There is still a lack of information. Doctors have less and less time. They make a diagnosis and then it is up to the patient.

Barnosell: Thank you. What I have experienced in all my fifteen years of shamanic life is that those from whom I have learned the most were people with no education, no university education, but who were sometimes able to cure tumors with their hands, for example. For me, a doctor used to science, this was just unbelievable. Of course, we are in a very complicated world. We live in a difficult society, we have more and more complexities, but we have to respect minorities, we have to respect people, different people. I have to say that therapists without a lot of titles are those who have taught me most. Since we doctors have university degrees we sometimes feel we are superior, but I think that in the future Western medicine has to evolve and integrate with other kinds of medicines. Of course, we have to work with professional people and I think that it is very important to unite our knowledge and abilities, but there are many seemingly ordinary people in this world who have very useful gifts. I always say that a healer I know is able to make a scan with his hands. That is something that really commands respect. Thank you.

Audience: I would like to thank you for organizing this symposium on Tibetan medicine. Thanks to the speakers, because I have really learned a lot.

Particularly, I would like to thank with all my heart Dr. Lobsang. I am a psychoanalyst. I would like to highlight two questions and two topics. First of all, Western society is obsessed with science. Everything needs to be scientific, but Western medical science is based on premises that were developed in the seventeenth century. So maybe we need to question whether we want to comply with the paradigm of medical science that was developed in the seventeenth century or challenge it. Secondly, I was really impressed by what Dr. Lobsang said: that before there weren't so many mental diseases. It is true that historically we have seen an evolution of society. But I would like to ask him: do you think that in the past we had fewer mental diseases due to the fact that society had a clearer structure, that there were some norms, that there were some clear parameters, that there were some clear social and spiritual relationships? Society had a very clear framework also for mental suffering. I would like to ask him what he thinks about the fact that we have many more mental diseases now than in the past.

Lobsang: I hope I understood the question correctly and I'll try to answer. If I have misunderstood you, please forgive me. When I say I like science, I do so according to my own view. If a person has great knowledge and uses it for positive purposes he will get wonderful results; but if such knowledge in used inappropriately or negatively, it can also create tremendously negative results. Science is like that: it can be used in a negative or in a positive way. But anyway science is still in an early stage; it's like a teenager. Through science we do sometimes have a lot of negative results. It depends on who is using scientific knowledge and how they are using it.

Ten or twenty years ago, if you wanted to explain something about a traditional medicine, like Tibetan medicine to a public audience, many people would not agree and would not accept it. If we mentioned Buddha, people would say, "Who or what is Buddha? Is Buddha a professor or a person or something like knowledge?" Such people have no idea. For us it is very difficult to explain or to prove in a concrete way. So, [modern] scientists became like a bridge to explain whatever Buddha taught, whatever traditional medicine says, whatever we have of this ancient knowledge. They translate our knowledge into modern language and introduce it to the new generations or new public audiences. So science became for us like a bridging language.

As I said before, if we use science in a positive way there are a lot of benefits related to how to treat disease and how to give facility to social life, human life. I like science when it is used in a positive way for these purposes.

Also, one of the main teachings of the Buddha was that you should not trust anything; you should check, you should test everything. If you find something is true, if there is some proof, then you can use it. Buddha said: "You do not even have to believe me; you shouldn't think you have to believe whatever I say because I am an enlightened being. It is important for you to check." So my point of view on science is the same as that of Buddha. He said testing everything brings a sort of logical proof. I follow the same path; that way I like. That is concrete knowledge. I also like that. Thank you very much.

Moragas (representing the conference organizers): I do not want to give a talk, but I would like to say that the logo we used for this conference is particularly nice. Chögyal Namkhai Norbu saw four hearts, four continents in this logo, and when someone asked who designed it he said it does not really matter, it is here. What I really wanted to communicate to you is that this event is a fruit, a product of the help of many people. I also did my part, and I think that it has worked very well. Sometimes there are many stressful moments when you organize an event, but I have to say that everybody, I cannot tell you all their names, but all of the people at the table, all the technicians, and everybody have been very helpful. We never had difficulties. Everybody put their heart into it. And that is why and how it really succeeded.

In life we always say: "If we had had more time..." but I think that we really managed to make the best out of our time and we can always improve. I would like to thank specifically Roberti di Sarsina because he contributed a lot of ideas, he gave us a lot of advice on what was working and was not working.

I would like to thank everybody who allowed us to have this event here. I would like to thank the speakers as well. They also put their heart into it. They gave us all of their knowledge, all their experience. I would also like to thank the moderators; they themselves could have given many talks, because they are really great professionals. Here they had a more anonymous function, but I would like to thank them because obviously their work is vital and they were also vital to this event. Also thanks to the technicians, to people who took care of the catering, of the logistics, and of the webcast.

I would like to add that since the conference was broadcast by webcast, people of different countries all over the world were following, not just us. We had sponsors who promoted the event, such as Santiveri, for example, and the Miralle Foundation, especially Benedetta [Tagliabue Miralle]. This is the beginning of a movement for us. We have created a specific webpage for this conference. There is an e-mail address, there will be links, and thus we hope to give you a chance to communicate and to talk about the event. We have recorded all the talks, so you can access to them all through the link that is on the program. Thank you.

Now Phuntsog Wangmo is going to talk about the Shang Shung Institute.

Wangmo: On behalf of the International Shang Shung Institute I just wanted to say thank you to everybody individually. Today in the audience we have three Shang Shung representatives. We have Vladimir from Shang Shung Russia, Aldo from Shang Shung Italy, which as I said earlier is our original base, and then myself. This is a beginning;

this is our first conference on how we can integrate. I am looking forward to having more of these conferences everywhere and to continuing our collaboration to try to bring benefit to sentient beings. So, I just want to say thank you everybody.

CLOSING

First of all I would like to thank you all for being here, and for having done this journey together with us in this event.

On behalf of the organization, I too would like to thank everyone who has contributed to the organization of this symposium. Above all I would like to thank Professor Chögyal Namkhai Norbu, who actually had the idea to organize this, he proposed this conference; and whenever he proposes something we try to really carry it out. We would also like to thank the Tibetan School of Medicine of Shang Shung Institute for their help and cooperation, especially the cooperation of Dr. Phuntsog, who was very kind, very helpful, and gave us all her support.

Now Professor Namkhai Norbu will close this event. He was also the one who opened it.

Professor Namkhai Norbu: I want to say thank you very much to everybody for participating in this meeting, especially all the organizers, and also the doctors from different fields and different places. This kind of conference is particularly meaningful, because millions of people all over the world face illness. But knowledge of medicine is also crucial for healthy living, for people who don't have the problem of illness.

This is why we need to have more open collaboration among various fields and traditions of curing, and not remain closed and limited. Otherwise we will not be able to seriously help people. So this meeting of ours is very important. We met together; you doctors talked for days about your experience and knowledge. We need to continue and develop this kind of meeting for the future. This will be positive not only for Tibetan medicine, which is just one of the many medical traditions we have on this globe. The main point is that we need open collaboration in this field.

So, again, I want to thank everyone, including those of you who are not doctors, but are interested and want to know what we are doing and what is happening. We must understand that everybody has body, speech, and mind, and we need to know how to live and do our best for our life and our health. This is something very much connected with the knowledge and science of medicine, and we will continue in this direction. Thank you.

Distribution of Diplomas:

As a gesture of thanks and a reminder of this meeting, we would like to present a certificate of appreciation to all participating doctors and moderators:
Dr. Carlos Ramos
Dr. Francisco Barnosell
Dr. Phuntsog Wangmo
Dr. Thomás Álvaro Naranjo

Dr. Thubten Phuntsok
Dr. Carmen Martínez
Dr. Eva Juan Linares
Dr. Teresa Herrerías
Dr. Ishar Dalmau
Ms. Neus Rodríguez
Ms. Eloisa Álvarez Centeno
Dr. Paolo Roberti Di Sarsina
Dr. Guillem Martí
Dr. Serjo Abanades
Dr. Estela A. Beale
Dr. Li Qilin
Dr. Lobsang Tenzin
Dr. Imma Nogués

And now we can take a photograph together.

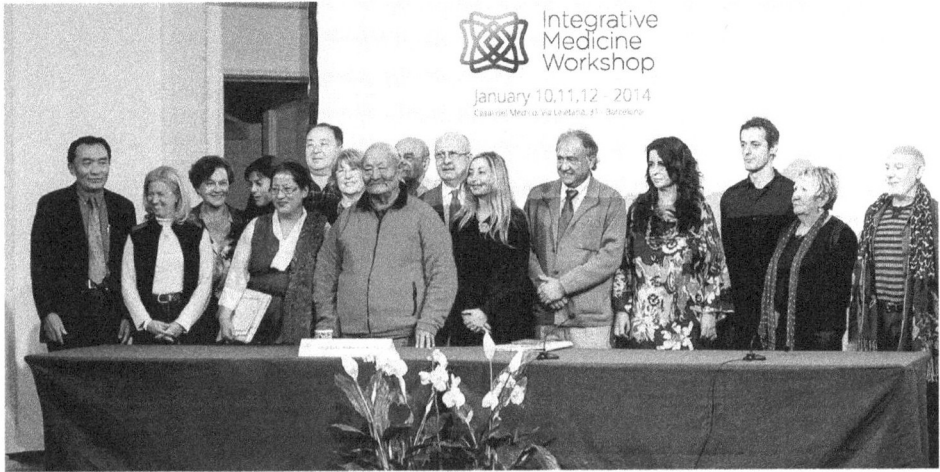

Group photo of conference participants.

www.ingramcontent.com/pod-product-compliance
Lightning Source LLC
Chambersburg PA
CBHW031925190326
41519CB00007B/412